A Clinical Guide to Pediatric
Weight Management and Obesity

A Clinical Guide to Pediatric Weight Management and Obesity

Sandra Gibson Hassink, M.D., F.A.A.P.

Assistant Professor of Pediatrics
Jefferson Medical College
Thomas Jefferson University
Philadelphia, Pennsylvania
Director, Weight Management Clinic
Alfred I. duPont Hospital for Children
Wilmington, Delaware

Wolters Kluwer | Lippincott Williams & Wilkins
Health
Philadelphia · Baltimore · New York · London
Buenos Aires · Hong Kong · Sydney · Tokyo

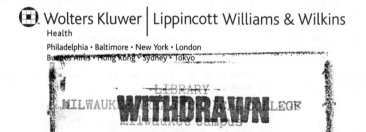

Acquisitions Editor: Sonya Seigafuse
Developmental Editor: Louise Bierig
Managing Editor: Ryan Shaw
Project Manager: Jennifer Harper
Manufacturing Coordinator: Kathleen Brown
Marketing Manager: Kimberly Schonberger
Creative Director: Doug Smock
Production Services: Nesbitt Graphics, Inc.
Printer: R.R. Donnelley, Crawfordsville

Printed in the USA

Library of Congress Cataloging-in-Publication Data

Hassink, Sandra Gibson.
  A guide to pediatric weight management and obesity / Sandra Gibson
Hassink.
  p. ; cm.
  Includes bibliographical references and index.
  ISBN-13: 978-0-7817-6480-3
  ISBN-10: 0-7817-6480-7
  1. Obesity in children--Prevention. 2. Overweight children
--Nutrition.   I. Title.
  [DNLM: 1. Obesity--prevention & control. 2. Adolescent.
  3. Child.   WD 210 H355g 2007]
  RJ399.C6H37 2007
  618.92'398--dc22
                                            2006027104

Care has been taken to confirm the accuracy of the information presented and to describe generally accepted practices. However, the authors, editors, and publisher are not responsible for errors or omissions or for any consequences from application of the information in this book and make no warranty, expressed or implied, with respect to the currency, completeness, or accuracy of the contents of the publication. Application of this information in a particular situation remains the professional responsibility of the practitioner.

The authors, editors, and publisher have exerted every effort to ensure that drug selection and dosage set forth in this text are in accordance with current recommendations and practice at the time of publication. However, in view of ongoing research, changes in government regulations, and the constant flow of information relating to drug therapy and drug reactions, the reader is urged to check the package insert for each drug for any change in indications and dosage and for added warnings and precautions. This is particularly important when the recommended agent is a new or infrequently employed drug.

Some drugs and medical devices presented in this publication have Food and Drug Administration (FDA) clearance for limited use in restricted research settings. It is the responsibility of the health care provider to ascertain the FDA status of each drug or device planned for use in their clinical practice.

To purchase additional copies of this book, call our customer service department at (800) 638-3030 or fax orders to (301) 223-2320. International customers should call (301) 223-2300.

Visit Lippincott Williams & Wilkins on the Internet: at LWW.com. Lippincott Williams & Wilkins customer service representatives are available from 8:30 am to 6 pm, EST.

10 9 8 7 6 5 4 3 2 1

Contents

Preface

Obesity represents the most common chronic illness of children and adolescents. Childhood obesity affects every age group from infancy to young adulthood and one quarter to one third of all pediatric patients. With the rapid onset of the "obesity epidemic," pediatric health care professionals are struggling to meet the clinical and educational demands required to care for obese patients and their families. Driven by the obesity epidemic, comorbidities previously seen only in adults are being diagnosed in children and adolescents, often requiring treatment by the pediatric practitioner.

Covered only briefly or not at all in medical school or residency training, obesity and obesity-related diseases constitute a new area of study for most pediatric health care providers. The mission of this book is to increase understanding of the epidemiology, pathophysiology, and effect of obesity in childhood and to address the obesity-related comorbidities in detail.

The initial chapters (Chapters 1–5) cover principles in obesity management, pathophysiology, and epidemiology, allowing the reader to develop an understanding of obesity in the context of gene-environment interaction, societal change, and the individual child and family. The following chapters (Chapters 6–14) focus on the pathophysiology, clinical manifestations, and treatment of the comorbidities of obesity. Topics include, among others, obesity-related genetic syndromes, type 2 diabetes and the metabolic syndrome, nonalcoholic steatohepatitis, hypertension and dyslipidemia, hypothalamic obesity, obesity-related orthopedic complications, and mental health issues. Each chapter discusses epidemiology, pathophysiology, clinical manifestations, and treatment, usually ending with a case presentation. Chapter 15 deals with specific emergencies related to obesity, and Chapter 16 offers strategies for treating the obese patient. The hope is that this book will add to the knowledge base of those who care for obese children and their families and provide help in managing this "new morbidity" in pediatrics.

This book is dedicated to my husband Bill,
my children Matthew, Stephen, and Alexa, with
gratitude for their unfailing enthusiasm and support,
and also to all those dedicated to the health of children
who have taught and mentored me over the years.

Acknowledgments

Special thanks go to the members of the Weight Management Team at the Alfred I. duPont Hospital for Children, who are dedicated to expanding their knowledge and skills in their efforts to give the best possible care to children with obesity and their families. Additional thanks are extended to the reviewers of this book, who have also shared their own subspecialty expertise with me: Laura Inselman, M.D., Bill Cochran, M.D., Vani Golparady, M.D., Sam Gidding, M.D., Daniel Doyle, M.D., Richard Bowen, M.D., Bruce Kaiser, M.D., Mena Scavena, M.D., and Marci Yonker, M.D.

A Clinical Guide to Pediatric Weight Management and Obesity

1

Introduction: Medical Management of Obesity

OBESITY

In ancient societies, obesity was traditionally seen as a sign of health and prosperity, because only prosperous individuals were assured of the ability to secure a stable, even abundant, supply of food in times of scarce resources. In addition, the ability to survive shifts in energy balance as a result of a variable food supply may have played a role in the selective survival of energy-efficient individuals. There has always been a crucial link between obesity and the individual's environment.

As the health of the population shifted, so did energy balance. In developing countries, improved nutrition, control of infectious diseases, and access to better living conditions have led to the ability to maintain increased energy stores as fat. In modern times, the rise of obesity in developing countries reflects this change in environmental conditions.

In the 1960s, for example, Chile experienced high maternal and infant mortality rates, along with a significant prevalence of infectious disease and malnutrition. In the succeeding 30 years, social programs were provided that increased the supply of food, improved educational systems and water and sanitation infrastructure, increased primary health care interventions, and lowered the unemployment rates. This meant that by the 1990s infant mortality had declined, mortality from communicable disease had decreased, and undernutrition was being replaced by obesity (1).

This pattern has been repeated in developing countries to such an extent that it, combined with the increase of obesity in more developed nations, has caused the World Health Organization to declare obesity a "worldwide epidemic" (2).

In developed countries, the trends driving the increase in obesity have not necessarily been the result of "positive" social and economic advancement. In the United

1

States, for instance, Native Americans have experienced one of the fastest increases in obesity rates (3). In particular, the Pima Indian tribe has been among the most studied examples of the rapid rise of obesity secondary to shifts in the environment (4). The concept of the "thrifty genotype" has been advanced to explain the tendency of a population that has traditionally been exposed to cycles of food scarcity to become obese in the face of a stable and abundant food source (5). In the past one to two generations, as diets shifted toward increased fat intake and lifestyles became more sedentary, the rates of obesity rose alarmingly in the Pima population. By way of explanation, the composition of the Pima Indian diets of 100 years ago consisted of approximately 70% to 80% carbohydrate, 8% to 12% fat, and 12% to 18% protein; the current Pima diet consists of approximately 47% carbohydrate, 35% fat, 15% protein, and 3% alcohol (6). Factors affecting food choices on Indian reservations have been cost, availability, and shelf life. Higher fat foods available on reservations are cheaper, and lack of refrigeration makes purchase of perishable items such as fruits and vegetables less likely (7). At the same time dietary patterns were changing, physical activity was decreasing, with Pima children spending more time watching television and being less involved in sports than white children (8).

In more affluent environments where choices are possible, people make choices dictated by the "built environment" (9). The sociocultural desire to save time and decrease exertion may be driving the changes in the physical environment (9). "With our intelligence, we've acquired the knowledge to change our environment at speeds that our natural, evolutionary abilities cannot adapt to" (E. Zerhouni) (9). In light of the fact that "genetically, we are designed to eat when we can, and rest when we don't have to be physically active" (J. Hill) (9), these sociocultural environmental changes are not congruent with our genetic programming.

CHILDHOOD GROWTH

Poor growth has always been associated with poor health. In a pediatric medicine text from 1853, physicians were instructed to observe the child's size as an indicator of health or disease.

> A child who has been healthy from its birth ought to have attained a certain average size and development at a certain age. If, on the contrary, it be much below the average size, if at three months it look like a newborn children, or at a year old like one of six months, it is very clear that something has acted to determine such slow and insufficient growth and it becomes the business of the practitioner to discover what the impeding cause has been (10).

Using growth charts to track the rate of weight and height gain has, until relatively recently, been focused on the child who is underweight or has slowing growth or "failure to thrive." This type of growth pattern has been the impetus to closely examine the physical, psychosocial, and environmental influences that affect the child. Parents and families also have viewed the child's size and growth as an indicator of health, and in many cultures, parents prefer larger children. In 1999, a study of urban and rural Chinese families revealed that an increase in weight in young children was perceived as a sign of health and prosperity (11).

THE BALANCE SHIFTS

The rising rates of obesity in all countries have been explained by a shift in energy balance caused by an increasingly sedentary lifestyle, greater consumption of non-nutritious high-calorie "junk food," increased eating frequency and portion size, and the emergence of television and computer use. The change in these environmental factors has not been hard to track and correlate with rising obesity rates in children. Actual causal links have been harder to establish. It is valuable to study attempts to analyze the trends that gave rise to shifts in population from underweight to overweight in an effort to understand the environmental forces acting on the population, which may have the potential to be changed.

In Chile, determinants of obesity were analyzed using data from a two-decade period between 1980 and 2000, when obesity increased at a rapid rate, with prevalence almost tripling. Environmental indicators, which relate to energy balance, were analyzed. Over this period, the mean caloric intake per day per person increased by 200 kcal, but this more than tripled when expressed as kilocalories per day per person living in poverty (1).

Two points may be made here. The first is that the daily increase of each 100 kcal beyond what is required to balance energy expenditure may be responsible for an approximate 10 lb per year weight gain in a person genetically susceptible to obesity; so, small amounts of caloric imbalance that occur consistently can account for substantial increases in weight. The second point is that food supplementation programs targeted to impoverished populations may have resulted in greater caloric imbalances at the same time that the energy expenditures were decreasing, resulting in a disproportionate weight gain. This is illustrated by data from the same study (1), which indicate that the numbers of cars, phones, and televisions in the population increased along with trends in the rise of sedentary behavior.

THE INTRAUTERINE ENVIRONMENT

Additional aspects of the interaction between the environment and the individual indicate that there may be susceptible periods in growth that sensitize the individual to obesity-promoting environments.

Young men whose mothers were exposed to undernutrition in the first and second trimesters of pregnancy during the Dutch famine of World War II were more likely to be obese than those whose mothers were exposed during the third trimester and those adults whose mothers were not undernourished (12).

Intrauterine growth may affect later body composition and deposition of adipose tissue. British men born with evidence of intrauterine growth retardation had greater waist-to-hip ratios for body mass index (BMI) than men of normal birth weight, indicating increased visceral fat deposition. Mexican and white Americans in the lowest third of birth weight had greater truncal fat than the highest third, which raises the possibility of an effect of intrauterine growth on body composition (13).

Diabetes in women during pregnancy has also been associated, in many studies, with an increased risk of diabetes and obesity in their children independent of maternal weight or infant birth weight (14). One hypothesis offered to explain this finding is that chronic hyperinsulinemia as a result of a hyperglycemic intrauterine environment might downregulate insulin receptors or post–insulin receptor signaling, giving rise to increasing insulin resistance in the child (15). Data from the National Health and Nutrition Examination Survey (NHANES) II for a sample of U.S. children between 2 and 47 months showed that babies born small for gestational age (SGA, birth weight <10th percentile) had a persistent deficit in lean body mass. At any given weight in this group, percent body fat was relatively higher for children who were SGA at birth (16).

In 1992, Hales and Barker (17) raised the possibility of the intrauterine environment's importance in "programming" a response to the nutritional environment later in life. Relative undernutrition in the intrauterine environment that causes a smaller than expected birth weight is associated with the development of obesity, diabetes, and cardiovascular disease in midlife. The mechanism for this increased risk is not known, but it raises the issue of the existence of vulnerable periods in growth and development that have a long-lasting effect on the response of the individual to the environment.

Infancy may be another vulnerable time in which rapid growth may predispose to later obesity. In a study of infant and childhood growth in an African American population, children who were in the highest growth percentiles at 4 months of age had a greater chance of being overweight by age 8 (18).

GENE-ENVIRONMENT INTERACTION

The "thrifty genotype" proposes that the genetics most suitable for survival in an energy-scarce environment of recurrent food shortages will cause weight gain in an energy-rich environment (5). Pérusse and Bouchard (19) have noted that "genotype-environment interactions arise when the response of a phenotype (e.g., fat mass) to environmental changes (e.g., dietary intervention) is modulated by the genotype of the individual." They further speculate that these effects may explain individual responses to dietary constituents and/or susceptibility to obesity-related comorbidity (19).

A study of the effect of overfeeding on twin pairs showed that the difference in fat storage between pairs was sixfold greater than within pairs, indicating that genetic characteristics are modulating in response to energy surplus. In an exercise study, twins were more alike in their response to negative energy balance than were individuals of different genotypes (19). In the same way, carriers of a specific polymorphism in the lipoprotein lipase gene were shown to gain more weight and body fat in response to overfeeding than noncarriers (20).

Individual susceptibility to energy imbalance increases in importance as the environment becomes more obesity promoting, the interaction between the environment and the individual determining who will become obese in a given environment.

Control of energy regulation has been proposed to reside within three distinct physiologic systems in the body: (a) the control of partitioning between protein and fat; (b) the nonspecific control of thermogenesis with afferent signals arising from food deprivation, nutrient deficiency, excess energy intake, and exposure to infection or cold stress; and (c) the adipose-specific control of thermogenesis, which is regulated by signals arising from the state of depletion of the adipose tissue fat stores (21).

The control of body energy partitioning operates during cycles of energy restriction (starvation) and energy abundance (refeeding). An individual's body composition dictates the proportion of protein and fat to be mobilized and used as fuel when starvation occurs and the proportion of deposition of protein and fat during refeeding (21). This explains why weight gain in obesity is due to an increase in both adipose tissue and lean body mass, the proportions of which vary in each individual (22). With the same excess caloric intake, then, an individual with a low partitioning characteristic will gain more fat and less protein than an individual with a high partitioning characteristic (21). This characteristic may be one of the major genetically determined physiologic variables in the development of obesity (21).

Nonspecific control of thermogenesis or diet-induced thermogenesis is regulated by the sympathetic nervous system and can be affected by energy supply, diet composition, nutrient deficiencies, ambient temperature, and psychological stress (21). This control system suppresses thermogenesis under conditions of energy scarcity, and the suppression is rapidly removed when food becomes available again. The system may have evolved as a mechanism for regulating the supply of essential nutrients rather than overall energy balance (23). For example, excess calories consumed from a poor diet in an effort to replace essential nutrients would trigger diet-induced thermogenesis to avoid excess weight gain. Individual differences in diet-induced thermogenesis are greater when high- or low-protein diets are overfed. Stock (23) maintains that this could provide a highly sensitive method for discriminating between those who are, in metabolic terms, resistant to obesity and those who are susceptible to it.

Adipose-specific thermogenesis is a process that causes a disproportionate deposition of fat relative to lean tissue in a cycle of weight recovery after energy scarcity (21). This mechanism is believed to have survival value because fat has a greater energy density and lower cost of maintenance than lean tissue and would enable an individual to rapidly build back an energy reserve for the next food shortage (21).

HEALTH AND DISEASE IN CHILDHOOD: A SHIFTING PARADIGM

In the early part of the 20th century, efforts to improve child health focused on vaccination, treatment of infectious disease and cancer, and improvement in nutrition. Obesity-related comorbidities were not in evidence. No physician in training 25 years ago expected to see a 12-year-old with type 2 diabetes or a teen with nonalcoholic hepatosteatosis. Obesity was just beginning to increase, and the obesity-related diseases hovered on the horizon. The obesity-related comorbidities that are discussed in this book represent "new morbidity" for children, which will require prevention efforts, intervention, and treatment strategies. Increased understanding of the pathophysiology, evolution, and treatment of these diseases can help physicians stem the rising tide of morbidity that threatens the health of children and adolescents.

REFERENCES

1. Kain J, Burrows R, Uauy R. Obesity trends in Chilean children and adolescents; basic determinants. In: Chen C, Dietz W, eds. *Obesity in childhood and adolescence,* Nutrition Workshop Series. Pediatric Program, Vol. 49. Nestec Ltd. Philadelphia: Vevey/Lippincott Williams & Wilkins; 2002:45–64.
2. World Health Organization. Global Strategy on Diet, Physical Activity and Health. http://www.who.int/dietphysicalactivity/publications/facts/obesity/en/
3. Story M, Evans M, Fabsitz RR, Clay TE, Holy Rock B, Broussard B. The epidemic of obesity in American Indian communities and the need for childhood obesity prevention programs. *Am J Clin Nutr.* 1999;69(4):747S–754S.
4. Tataranni PA, Harper IT, Snitker S, Del Parigi A, Vozarova B, Bunt J, Bogardus C, Ravussin E. Body weight gain in free-living Pima Indians: effect of energy intake vs. expenditure. *Int J Obes Relat Metab Disord.* 2003;27(12):1578–1584.
5. Neel JV. Diabetes mellitus: a "thrifty" genotype rendered detrimental by progress. *Am J Hum Genet.* 1962;14:353–362.
6. Boyce VL, Swinburn BA. The traditional Pima diet: composition and adaptation for use in a dietary intervention study. *Diabetes Care.* 1993;16(1):369–371.
7. Ballew C, White L, Strauss K, Benson L, Mendlein J, Mokdad A. Intake of nutrients and food sources of nutrients among the Navajo: findings from the Navajo Health and Nutrition Survey. *J Nutr.* 1997;127(10 suppl):2085S–2093S.
8. Fontvieille A, Kriska A, Ravussin E. Decreased physical activity in Pima Indians compared with Caucasian children. *Int J Obes Relat Metab Disord.* 1993;17(8):445–452.
9. Spotswood S. NIH highlights link between obesity and environment. *US Medicine,* July 2004. Available at: http://www.usmedicine.com/article.cfm?articleID=902&issueID=64 (accessed July 14, 2006).
10. Forsyth Meigs J. *Practical treatise on the diseases of children,* 3rd ed., carefully revised. Philadelphia: Lindsay and Blankiston; 1858.
11. Ma G. Environmental factors leading to pediatric obesity in the developing world. In: Chen C, Dietz W, eds. *Obesity in childhood and adolescence.* Nestle Nutrition Workshop Series. Pediatric Program, Vol. 49. Nestec Ltd. Philadelphia: Vevey/Lippincott Williams & Wilkins; 2002:195–206.
12. Ravelli GP, Stein ZA, Susser MW. Obesity in young men after famine exposure in utero and early infancy. *N Engl J Med.* 1976;295(7):349–353.
13. Jackson AA, Langley-Evans SC, McCarthy HD. Nutritional influences in early life upon obesity and body proportions. *Ciba Found Symp.* 1996;201:118–137, 188–193.
14. Whitaker RC, Dietz WH. Role of prenatal environment in the development of obesity. *J Pediatr.* 1998;132(5):768–776.
15. Singhal A, Lanigan J, Lucas A. Early origins of obesity. In: Chen C, Dietz W, eds. *Obesity in childhood and adolescence.* Nestle Nutrition Workshop Series. Pediatric Program. Vol. 49. Nestec Ltd. Philadelphia: Vevey/Lippincott Williams & Wilkins; 2002:83–97.
16. Hediger ML, Overpeck MD, Kuczmarski RJ, , McGlynn A, Maurer KR, Davis WW. Muscularity and fatness of infants and young children born small or large for gestational age. *Pediatrics.* 1998; 102(5):E60.
17. Hales CN, Barker DJ. Type 2 (non-insulin dependent) diabetes mellitus: the thrifty phenotype hypothesis. *Diabetologia.* 1992;35(7):595–601.
18. Stettler N, Kumanyika SK, Katz SH, Zemel BS, Stallings VA. Rapid weight gain during infancy and obesity in young adulthood in a cohort of African Americans. *Am J Clin Nutr.* 2003;77(6): 1374–1378.
19. Pérusse L, Bouchard C. Gene-diet interaction in obesity. *Am Clin Nutr.* 2000;72(5 suppl): 1285S–1290S.
20. Bouchard C, Dionne FT, Chagnon M, Moreel JF, Pérusse L. DNA sequence variation in the lipoprotein lipase (LPL) gene and obesity. *FASEB J.* 1994;8:923(abst).
21. Dulloo AG, Jacquet J. Toward understanding the genetic basis of human susceptibility to obesity: a systemic approach. In: Chen C, Dietz W, eds. *Obesity in childhood and adolescence.* Nestle Nutrition Workshop Series. Pediatric Program, Vol. 49. Nestec Ltd. Philadelphia: Vevey/Lippincott Williams & Wilkins; 2002:143–161.
22. Forbes GB. Lean body mass-body fat interrelationship in humans. *Nutr Rev.* 1987;45(8):225–231.
23. Stock MJ. Gluttony and thermogenesis revisited. *Int J Obes Relat Metab Disord.*1999;23:1105–1117.

2

Epidemiology of
Childhood Obesity

THE EPIDEMIC OF OBESITY

The rapid rise in obesity among children and adults has been declared a worldwide epidemic (1). Obesity is increasing at an alarming rate in both developed and developing countries. Similar factors are operating across the globe to raise obesity rates in children (2):

- Increases in economic welfare
- Stability of the food supply
- Rising standards of living
- Increases in energy-dense diets
- Television ownership
- Increase in sedentary leisure time

> Alterations in global, national, community, family, and childhood nutrition and activity patterns have been rapid and pervasive.

Transitions in patterns of physical activity and nutrition have caused rates of obesity to approach those of malnutrition for the first time (3). Unfortunately, changes in systems of nutritional support, the activity environment, and leisure activities have yet to stop the increase in children's weight.

SHIFTS IN THE POPULATION

The percentage of adults who are at a healthy weight has declined progressively over the past two decades (Fig. 2.1) (4), with a corresponding increase in overweight and obesity. Since 1980, adult overweight has risen by 17.8% and obesity by 16% (4).

Children and adolescents have paralleled this trend (Fig. 2.2) (4). Obesity has risen by 10.2% from 1980 to 2000 in 12- to 19-year-olds and by 9.3% in 6- to 11-year-olds (4).

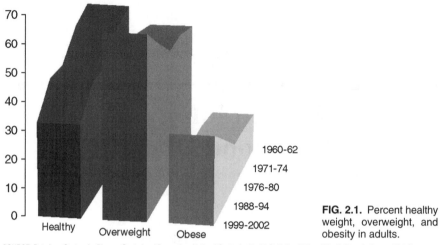

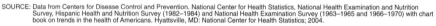

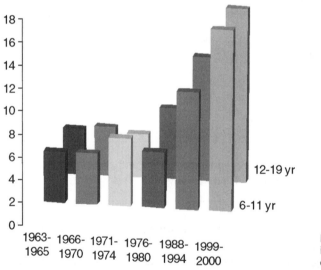

FIG. 2.1. Percent healthy weight, overweight, and obesity in adults.

SOURCE: Data from Centers for Disease Control and Prevention. National Center for Health Statistics, National Health Examination and Nutrition Survey, Hispanic Health and Nutrition Survey (1982–1984) and National Health Examination Survey (1963–1965 and 1966–1970) with chart book on trends in the health of Americans. Hyattsville, MD: National Center for Health Statistics; 2004.

FIG. 2.2. Percent obesity in children and adolescents.

SOURCE: Data from Centers for Disease Control and Prevention. National Center for Health Statistics, National Health Examination and Nutrition Survey, Hispanic Health and Nutrition Survey (1982–1984) and National Health Examination Survey (1963–1965 and 1966–1970) with chart book on trends in the health of Americans. Hyattsville, MD: National Center for Health Statistics; 2004.

In the past 25 years, major shifts toward obesity have occurred in all populations. Genetic predisposition to obesity clearly exists; for example, children of obese parents (one or both) have a much greater incidence of obesity (5). In fact, a child whose parent or parents are obese has only a 10% chance of having a normal weight by the end of adolescence (Fig. 2.3) (5).

Genetics alone, however, cannot explain the epidemic proportions of the obesity problem. A gene-environment interaction is clearly at work. One explanation is called the "thrifty genotype hypothesis" (6). For most of human history, populations

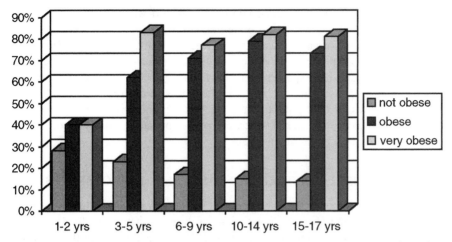

FIG. 2.3. Prevalence of obesity in young adults with at least one obese parent. (Data from Whitaker RC, Wright JA, Pepe MS, Seidel KD, Dietz WH. Predicting obesity in young adulthood from childhood and parental obesity. *N Engl J Med.* 1997;337:869–873, with permission.)

were dependent on a problematic food supply—times of plenty alternating with scarcity. Survival was predicated on the ability of an individual to conserve energy stores and minimize energy expenditure. In this situation, the theory states, a population would eventually develop in which individuals "programmed" for cycles of "feast or famine" with energy-efficient metabolisms would predominate. In recent history, food has become plentiful and energy expenditure has decreased.

Populations and individuals who are energy efficient now have excess calories to store as adipose tissue, and obesity is the result.

This theory may also explain why the susceptibility to obesity seems to differ between ethnic populations who developed under different conditions of energy availability. Developing nations are also experiencing this phenomenon as improved health status, food availability, and decreased energy expenditure are accelerating the societal transition from high rates of malnutrition to obesity.

Predisposition to obesity may also be increasing on an individual level. It is true that obesity "runs in families," indicating traditional inheritance patterns for energy regulation. However, the concept of programming an individual's response to the environment has recently emerged in the "thrifty phenotype" hypothesis. Hales and Barker (7) noted that older individuals with increased rates of diabetes had smaller than average birth weights. Reduced birth weight has also been associated with increased insulin resistance (8), cardiovascular disease, and increased central adiposity (9). In this theory, infants who had a relatively energy-restricted intrauterine environment altered their genetic programming accordingly. In other words, these infants were responding to an environment of scarcity by becoming more energy efficient. However, when these infants are born into an energy-rich environment, their intrauterine adaptations work against them; they develop central obesity and susceptiblity to later obesity-related comorbidities (10).

The intrauterine environment also plays a critical role at the other end of the birth weight spectrum. Infants born to diabetic or obese mothers tend to be larger than normal. These infants are exposed to higher levels of glucose *in utero* and mount a greater insulin response, and this may alter insulin receptor expression and change insulin sensitivity to the extrauterine environment (11). This programming increases their risk for later obesity and diabetes, thereby perpetuating this cycle of altered response to the energy environment (12).

SUSCEPTIBLE POPULATIONS—ADVERSE ENVIRONMENTS

Obesity affects minority populations disproportionately. Rates of obesity among African American and Hispanic populations are greater than those for Caucasian children and have escalated more rapidly (Fig. 2.4) (4). The reasons for this disparity are not entirely clear.

Obesity-promoting influences may be more intense in disadvantaged and ethnic minorities. For example, African American and Hispanic children watch more television, movies, and videos than Caucasian children, as do children from low-income families of all ethnic groups. (13). The complexity of the interaction between ethnicity and obesity is illustrated in the different explanatory models (14) for fruit and vegetable consumption among white, African American, and Hispanic adults of similar low to moderate economic status. Among white adults, having a garden, being single with no child, or being married with a young child was positively associated with fruit and vegetable consumption. Among African Americans, fruit and vegetable consumption was associated with a higher educational level. Hispanic adults reported that liking fruits and vegetables as a child, changing their diet for health reasons, and having food skills were positively associated with fruit and vegetable consumption (14).

Sometimes, even well-intentioned services may inadvertently encourage obesity. The National School Lunch and National School Breakfast Program, for example, is used more by low-income and minority children (13). Tables 2.1 and 2.2 list the food composition of school-provided breakfast and lunch (15).

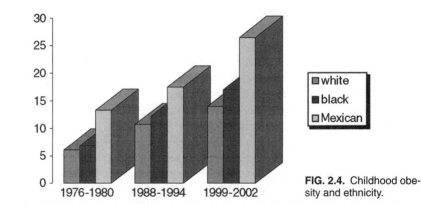

FIG. 2.4. Childhood obesity and ethnicity.

SOURCE: Data from Centers for Disease Control and Prevention. National Center for Health Statistics, National Health Examination and Nutrition Survey, Hispanic Health and Nutrition Survey (1982–1984) and National Health Examination Survey (1963–1965 and 1966–1970) with chart book on trends in the health of Americans. Hyattsville, MD: National Center for Health Statistics; 2004.

TABLE 2.1. *Minimum nutrient and calorie levels for school lunches—nutrient standard menu planning approaches (school week averages)*

	Minimum requirements			Optional
Nutrients and energy allowances	Preschool	Grades K–3	Grades 4–12	Grades 7–12
Energy allowances (calories)	517	633	785	825
Total fat (as a percentage of actual total food energy)	No more than 30% of total calories	No more than 30% of total calories	No more than 30% of total calories	No more than 30% of total calories
Saturated fat (as a percentage of actual total food energy)	Less than 10% of total calories	Less than 10% of total calories	Less than 10% of total calories	Less than 10% of total calories
RDA for protein (g)	7	9	15	16
RDA for calcium (mg)	267	267	370	4,000
RDA for iron (mg)	3.3	3.3	4.2	4.5
RDA for vitamin A (RE)	150	200	285	300
RDA for vitamin C (mg)	14	15	17	18

RDA, recommended dietary allowance.

1, The Dietary Guidelines recommend that after 2 years of age "...children should gradually adopt a diet that, by about 5 years of age, contains no more than 30 percent of calories from fat"; 2, total fat not to exceed 30% over a school week; 3, saturated fat less than 10% over a school week (15).

Data from http://www.fns.usda.gov/cnd/menu/menu.planning.approaches.for.lunches.doc.

TABLE 2.2. *Minimum nutrient and calorie levels for school breakfasts—nutrient standard menu planning approaches (school week averages)*

	Minimum requirements		Optional
Nutrients and energy allowances	Preschool	Grades K–12	Grades 7–12
Energy allowances (calories)	388	554	618
Total fat (as a percentage of actual total food energy)	No more than 30% of total calories	No more than 30% of total calories	No more than 30% of total calories
Saturated fat (as a percentage of actual total food energy)	Less than 10% of total calories	Less than 10% of total calories	Less than 10% of total calories
RDA for protein (g)	5	10	12
RDA for calcium (mg)	200	257	300
RDA for iron (mg)	2.5	3	3.4
RDA for Vitamin A (RE)	113	197	225
RDA for Vitamin C (mg)	11	13	14

RDA, recommended dietary allowance.

1, The Dietary Guidelines recommend that after 2 years of age "...children should gradually adopt a diet that, by about 5 years of age, contains no more than 30 percent of calories from fat"; 2, total fat not to exceed 30% over a school week; 3, saturated fat less than 10% over a school week; 4, "In order to be reimbursed, the snacks must contain at least two different components of the following four: a serving of fluid milk; a serving of meat or meat alternate; a serving of vegetable(s) or fruit(s) or full strength vegetable or fruit juice; a serving of whole grain or enriched bread or cereal" (15).

Data from http://www.fns.usda.gov/cnd/breakfast/Menu/sbp-planning-approaches.doc.

Although caloric intake represents a gross estimation of energy need (depending on activity and growth requirements), it is easy to see that a 5-year-old child eating breakfast and lunch at school would have already consumed 900 kcal before arriving home, not counting a midmorning snack, which might be 100 to 200 kcal. An average kilocalorie intake, assuming more than 60 minutes of activity per day, is 1,600 kcal/ day (16); dinner, snacks, and beverage intake would need to be limited to 500 to 700 kcal to meet this goal. It is easy to see how energy imbalance can occur. In addition, the minimum energy content of school meals is not varied across the age range from elementary school to high school, despite changes in energy needs.

Conditions that limit activity may be more common in minority populations and among low socioeconomic groups. For example, in 2003, 15.3% of African American adults had chronic conditions that limited activity compared with 10.2% of Hispanic individuals and 11.8% of white adults (4). The impact of poverty is significant and additive: The percentage of persons in poverty with chronic, activity-limiting conditions rose to 26.1% for African Americans, to 15.5% for Hispanic adults, and to 26.2% for white individuals (4). The effect on children is not known; however, the impressive limitation of activity among family members in minority and disadvantaged populations may play a role in activity availability in the family setting for these children.

SHIFTS IN THE ENVIRONMENT

The more "obesity promoting" the environment becomes, the higher the rate of obesity in the population.

Obesity-promoting trends include:

- Increased portion sizes
- Higher rates of sweetened beverage consumption
- Increased television and screen time
- Increased snacking
- Decreased physical activity in schools, neighborhoods, and communities

Portion Size

Portion sizes have increased dramatically from 1977 to 1996; soft drinks, salty snacks, french fries, and desserts are just some examples of food that are offered in larger amounts both inside and outside the home (17). Table 2.3 and Figure 2.5 illustrate the increases in snack food, fast food, and soft drink kilocalories over a 20-year period in the United States (17).

Increasing portion size has several implications. More food is offered at each meal and snack, irrespective of energy expenditure, increased portions are often seen as "value added" in terms of food dollars spent, and expectations may be raised

TABLE 2.3. *Increases in snack and fast food kilocalories over a 20-year period in the United States*

Salty snacks	Soft drinks	French fries
1977–1978 132 kcal	1977–1978 316 kcal	1977–1978 188 kcal
1989–1991 199 kcal	1989–1991 334 kcal	1989–1991 247 kcal
1994–1996 225 kcal	1994–1996 357 kcal	1994–1996 256 kcal

Data from Nielsen SJ, Popkin BM. Patterns and trends in food portion sizes, 1977–1998. *JAMA.* 2003;289(4):450–453.

for larger servings at home. In terms of children, extra-sized portions offered in restaurants and fast food establishments are uniform and not tailored to the individual age or activity level of the child.

Excess Snacking

The excess calories represented by snack food, french fries, and soft drinks can add up to marked increases in weight over time. For example, one extra serving of chips (salty snack food) per day in excess of the calories needed would have resulted in a weight gain of 13 lb/ year in 1977 and 23 lb/ year in 1994. Figure 2.6 illustrates the pounds per year of weight gain resulting from one extra serving of salty snack food, french fries, or a soft drink in excess of energy expenditure (17).

Television

Television viewing has also increased over time and has been associated with higher rates of obesity. In a survey of children from 1988 to 1994, it was found that more than one half of 8- to 16-years-old watched more than 2 hours of television per day. Many children were watching more than 5 hours per day, and the same study found that "on the average, 17% of non-Hispanic black children watched 5 hours or more a day, whereas only 9% of Latino American and 6% of non-Hispanic white children watched television for 5 or more hours a day" (18).

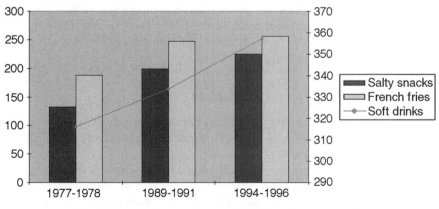

FIG. 2.5. Increase in snack and soft drink kilocalories per portion.

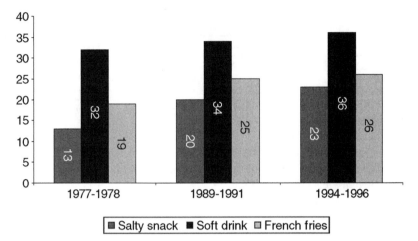

FIG. 2.6. Pounds of weight gain per year for one extra serving per day. (Data from Nielsen SJ, Popkin BM. Patterns and trends in food portion sizes, 1977–1998. *JAMA*. 2003;289(4): 450–453.)

> Children are a vulnerable population in the current nutrition and activity environment.

They encounter high-calorie foods at home, schools, daycare, and community centers and in restaurants and fast food establishments. They are a target group for marketing and advertising aimed at snack foods and sugared beverages. Families are busy and under stress, and are often making nutrition and activity choices "on the run." Moreover, children are being afforded little opportunity for activity in school, with declining physical education and recess periods and after school programs aimed at homework completion instead of outdoor time. Parents and families are the interface between the child and environment but may often not have the knowledge or necessary parenting skills to combat the influences acting on their children. Figure 2.7 shows the complexity of the interactions facing parents, families, and pediatricians in combating the obesity epidemic.

COMORBIDITY

The rising rates of obesity are the harbinger of increased morbidity and mortality for a generation of children who, for the first time in a century, may have a shorter life expectancy than their parents.

This book will address, in depth, obesity-related comorbidities. Some examples of obesity-related comorbidities—diabetes, nonalcoholic steatohepatitis, slipped capital femoral epiphysis, and pseudotumor cerebri—are highlighted in the following discussion.

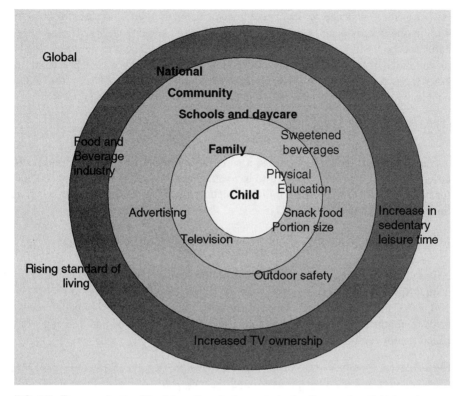

FIG. 2.7. The complexity of the interactions facing parents, families, and pediatricians in combating the obesity epidemic.

Diabetes

The lifetime risk of diabetes is now estimated to be 1 in 3 for boys and 2 in 5 for girls born in the year 2000 (19). Along with the increased lifetime risk for diabetes, the prevalence of type 2 diabetes in children has been reported to range from 4.1 per 1,000 in 12- to 19-year-old children in the United States (20) up to 50.9 per 1,000 in 15- to 19-year-olds in the high-risk Pima Indian population (21). Worldwide, the number of individuals with diabetes has tripled since 1985 (22).

Impaired glucose tolerance is a precursor to type 2 diabetes and is increased in obesity. In a study of obese children referred to a hospital clinic, Sinha et al. (23) found impaired glucose tolerance in 25% of the 55 children aged 4 to 10 years and 21% of 112 obese adolescents 11 to 18 years old, along with 4 adolescents who had previously undiagnosed diabetes.

Nonalcoholic Steatohepatitis

Nonalcoholic steatohepatitis (NASH) is another significant comorbidity of obesity, previously seen in adults, which has appeared in children and adolescents.

NASH has a prevalence of 3% in the general population and increases to 20% to 40% in obese individuals. Cirrhosis occurs in 25% of adults with NASH, and these patients account for up to 10% of liver-related deaths (24). The prevalence of NASH in childhood is not yet known. Nonalcoholic fatty liver disease, a precursor to NASH, has a prevalence of 2.6% in Japanese children (25). In a study from Italy, nonalcoholic fatty liver disease was found in 52.8% of obese children (26).

Slipped Capital Femoral Epiphysis

Slipped capital femoral epiphysis, a comorbidity of obesity unique to the pediatric population, has been reported to have an annual incidence of 2.22 per 100,000 for boys and 0.76 per 100,000 for girls in a study from Japan. This incidence is five times higher than that in 1976 (27).

Pseudotumor Cerebri

Pseudotumor cerebri is more common in obese than in normal weight children. In a study from Nova Scotia, the annual incidence in children was found to be 0.9 per 100,000. Cases were 2.7 times more likely in girls and twice as likely in adolescents (28). In another study, obesity was found in 29% of children and adolescents with pseudotumor cerebri (29).

Health care providers are at the epicenter of the obesity epidemic.

Prevention is critical, and every practitioner should have a strategy for encouraging healthy eating and activity habits in families and children at every health encounter. However, many children are already overweight or obese. These are the children and families who need our urgent attention. Intervention to prevent the development of comorbidities, treatment of existing comorbidity, and reversal of obesity whenever possible are critical tasks that cannot wait.

REFERENCES

1. Lobstein T, Baur L, Uauy R; IASO International Obesity TaskForce. Obesity in children and young people: a crisis in public health. *Obes Rev.* 2004;(suppl 1):4–104.
2. Wang Y, Monteiro C, Popkin BM. Trends of obesity and underweight in older children and adolescents in the United States, Brazil, China, and Russia. *Am J Clin Nutr.* 2002;75(6):971–977.
3. Rodgers A, Ezzati M, Vander Hoorn S, Lopez AD, Lin RB, Murray CJ; Comparative Risk Assessment Collaborating Group. Distribution of major health risks: findings from the Global Burden of Disease Study. *PLoS Med* 2004;1(1):e27.
4. Centers for Disease Control and Prevention. National Center for Health Statistics, National Health Examination and Nutrition Survey, Hispanic Health and Nutrition Survey (1982-1984) and National Health Examination Survey (1963-1965 and 1966-1970) with chart book on trends in the health of Americans. Hyattsville, MD: National Center for Health Statistics; 2004.

5. Whitaker RC, Wright JA, Pepe MS, Seidel KD, Dietz WH. Predicting obesity in young adulthood from childhood and parental obesity. *N Engl J Med.* 1997;337(13):869–873.
6. Neel JV. Diabetes mellitus: a "thrifty" genotype rendered detrimental by "progress"? *Am J Hum Genet.* 1962;14:353–362.
7. Hales CN, Barker DJ. The thrifty phenotype hypothesis. *Br Med Bull.* 2001;60:5–20.
8. Veening MA, Van Weissenbruch MM, Delemarre-Van De Wall HA. Glucose tolerance, insulin sensitivity and insulin secretion in children born small for gestational age. *J Clin Endocrinol Metab.* 2002;87(10):4657–4661.
9. Oken E, Gillman MW. Fetal origins of obesity. *Obes Res.* 2003;11:496–506.
10. Valdez R, Athens MA, Thompson GH, Bradshaw BH, Stern MP. Birthweight and adult health outcomes in a biethnic population in the U.S. *Diabetologia.* 1994 Jun;37(6):624–631.
11. Freinkel N. Of pregnancy and progeny (Banting lecture 1980). *Diabetes.* 1980;29:1023–1035.
12. Dabelea D, Petitt DJ. Intrauterine diabetic environment confers risks for type 2 diabetes mellitus and obesity in the offspring, in addition to genetic susceptibility. *J Pediatr Endocrinol Metab.* 2001;14(8):1085–1091.
13. Kumanyika S, Grier S. Targeting interventions for ethnic minority and low-income populations. *Future Child.* 2006;16(1):187–207.
14. Devine CM, Wolfe WS, Frongillo EA, Bisogni CA. Life-course events and experiences; association with fruit and vegetable consumption in 3 ethnic groups. *J Am Diet Assoc.*1999; 99(3):309–314.
15. http://teamnutrition.usda.gov/Resources/menuplanner_chapter2.pdf (accessed July 14, 2006).
16. http://www.mypyramid.gov/mypyramid/results.html?age=5&gender=male&activity=active (accessed July 14, 2006).
17. Nielsen SJ, Popkin BM. Patterns and trends in food portion sizes, 1977–1998. *JAMA.* 2003;289(4): 450–453.
18. Crespo CJ, Smit E, Troiano RP, Bartlett SJ, Macera C, Andersen RE. Television watching, energy intake and obesity in US children: results from the Third National Health and Nutrition Examination Survey, 1988-1994. *Arch Pediatr Adolesc Med.* 2001;155(3):360–365.
19. Narayan KM, Boyle JP, Thompson TJ, Sorensen SW, Williamson DF. Lifetime risk for diabetes mellitus in the United States. *JAMA.* 2003;290:1884–1890.
20. American Diabetes Association. Type 2 diabetes in children and adolescents. *Diabetes Care.* 2000;23(3):381–389.
21. Fagot-Campagna A, Pettitt DJ, Engelgau MM, Ríos Burrows N, Geiss LS, Valdez R, Beckles GL, Saaddine J, Gregg EW, Williamson DF, Narayan KM. Type 2 diabetes among North American children and adolescents: an epidemiological review and a public health perspective. *J Pediatr.* 2000;136(5): 664–672.
22. Bloomgarden ZT. Type 2 diabetes in the young: the evolving epidemic. *Diabetes Care.* 2004; 27(4): 998–1010.
23. Sinha R, Fisch G, Teague B, Tamborlane WV, Banyas B, Allen K, Savoye M, Rieger V, Taksali S, Barbetta G, Sherwin RS, Caprio S. Prevalence of impaired glucose tolerance among children and adolescents with marked obesity. *N Engl J Med.* 2002;346:802–810.
24. Youssef WI, McCullough AJ. Steatohepatitis in obese individuals. *Best Pract Res Clin Gastroenterol.* 2002;16(5):733–747.
25. Tominaga K, Kurata JH, Chen YK, Fujimoto E, Miyagawa S, Abe I, Kusano Y. Prevalence of fatty liver in Japanese children and relationship to obesity: an epidemiological ultrasonographic survey. *Dig Dis Sci.* 1995;40(9):2002–2009.
26. Franzese A, Vajro P, Argenziano A, Puzziello A, Iannucci MP, Saviano MC, Brunetti M, Rubino A. Liver involvement in obese children. Ultrasonography and liver enzyme levels at diagnosing and during follow-up in an Italian population. *Dig Dis Sci.* 1997;42(7):1438–1442.
27. Noguchi Y, Sakamaki T. Multicenter Study Committee of the Japanese Pediatric Orthopaedic Association Epidemiology and demographics of slipped capital femoral epiphysis in Japan: a multicenter study by the Japanese Paediatric Orthopaedic Association. *J Orthop Sci.* 2002;7(6):610–617.
28. Gordon K. Pediatric pseudotumor cerebri: descriptive epidemiology. *Can J Neurol Sci.* 1997;24(3): 219–221.
29. Scott IU, Siatkowski RM, Eneyni M, Brodsky MC, Lam BL. Idiopathic intracranial hypertension in children and adolescents. *Am J Ophthalmol.* 1997;124(2):253–255.

3

Pathophysiology of Obesity

Obesity has become a central theme in pediatric medicine. The impact of the obesity epidemic is felt in both the number of children affected and the rising rates of obesity-related comorbidities. This chapter reviews some highlights of obesity pathophysiology so the reader can begin to develop an increased understanding of pediatric obesity and effective prevention, early intervention, and treatment strategies.

ETIOLOGY

Obesity in childhood is a heterogeneous disease with unique weight gain trajectories, environmental triggers, and pathophysiologic responses.

> Every obese child and family has individual genetic, behavioral, relational, environmental, and physiologic characteristics that contribute to the development and maintenance of excess adiposity.

There may also be critical periods of susceptibility to obesity during the child's growth that make them especially vulnerable to obesity-promoting influences. Understanding the factors contributing to the cause of obesity may shed light on effective methods of treatment and enable the practitioner to help children and families make necessary lifestyle changes aimed toward weight loss.

Obesity is clearly a result of gene-environment interaction. The epidemic can be seen as an ever-worsening interplay of environmental factors overlying a continuum of genetic responsiveness. This interplay is even more complex when the impact of the intrauterine environment is taken into consideration. For instance, the risk for obesity and diabetes increases for children born to mothers who had diabetes during pregnancy (1).

In a study of middle-aged adults, Barker (2,3) found that adults who were small for gestational age newborns were at increased risk for obesity, diabetes, and hypertension. This finding points to the long-standing effect of environmental change when it occurs during a susceptible developmental period. The term "developmental plasticity" has been used to describe "the ability of a single genotype to produce more than one type of structure, physiologic state, or behavior in response to biologic conditions" (4). Infants who were exposed to cigarette smoke while *in utero,* one of the causes of intrauterine growth restriction, are at increased risk for obesity as well (5), the supposition being that the altered intrauterine environment also altered their susceptibility to later weight gain. A maternal diet high in carbohydrate early in pregnancy and low in protein late in pregnancy has also been associated with reduced placental weight and birth weight (6). Maternal hypertension, a risk for lower birth weight, can also reduce the ability of the placenta to transfer energy to the fetus (7), possibly adding to the infant's cumulative risk for later obesity.

The theory that altering the "programming" (8) of a fetus in the intrauterine environment may result in later changes in how the child responds to the environment represents a fundamental shift in thinking about what constitutes predisposition for later obesity. The mechanisms affecting the intrauterine environment and subsequent changes in individual response are not completely understood. It is hypothesized that an infant exposed to an energy-restricted intrauterine environment alters mechanisms of energy balance in preparation for a similarly restricted extrauterine environment. For example, under conditions of energy restriction *in utero,* fetal protein breakdown and amino acid utilization increase to maintain energy homeostasis at the expense of reducing energy required for growth (9). After birth, exposure to an energy-rich environment of "plenty" results in a "mismatch" between genetic programming for an environment of scarcity and the actual environmental experience of the infant. This mismatch leads to the accumulation of adipose tissue (10,11).

Intrauterine effects of diabetes or impaired glucose tolerance can also influence the future risk of obesity and diabetes. Increased exposure of the fetus to glucose, as occurs when the pregnant woman is diabetic, results in greater insulin production by the fetus and greater deposition of adipose tissue (1). Parental obesity, also a risk for later obesity, may reflect both genetic and environmental influences as well as psychobehavioral effects on eating and activity. Whitaker et al. (12) has shown that the risk of obesity when one or both parents are obese increases markedly as childhood advances.

Shared predisposition and shared environment mandate that prevention, intervention, and treatment efforts are targeted toward family-based change.

ENERGY INTAKE

Energy intake can be affected by multiple factors that represent the complex interaction between the external environment and the internal interplay of energy stores, central nervous system feedback, and psychological predisposition. The interface between the individual and the environment when food is readily available is modulated by hunger and satiety (Table 3.1).

TABLE 3.1. *Influence on energy intake*

Hunger	Psychological states	Visual cues
Satiety	Depression	Social expectations
Palatability	Anxiety	Social situations
Food availability	Reaction to stress	
Emotions		

Hunger

Hunger is the *internal* experience of a desire to eat. The child's expression of hunger is often the driving force behind parent-child interactions involving food. A variety of internal and external cues may trigger hunger (13), and awareness of these triggers may allow parents to respond with a solution to the underlying cause rather than with food.

- The pleasure of eating
- Emotional states of anxiety
- Depression
- Stress
- Social cues
- Sensory cues
- Boredom
- Environmental cues
- Timing

Appetite, on the other hand, has been defined as "the internal driving force for the search, choice and ingestion of food" (13). Appetite can also be thought of as the *external* expression of hunger. Blundell (14) breaks appetite down into an interaction between psychological events and behavior, peripheral physiology, and the central nervous system (CNS).

These three systems operate in the equation of energy balance and dysfunction and at any level can alter energy intake. Studies have shown that food intake increases as taste becomes more pleasant (15). In studies with rats, greater availability of highly palatable foods increases intake, resulting in what Tordorff calls "obesity by choice" (16). Pleasant taste and aversion to tastes have been linked to the amygdala and orbital frontal cortex (17).

Feedback from the gastrointestinal tract can also affect the experience of hunger and appetite. Ghrelin, a 28-amino-acid acylated peptide, is the endogenous ligand for the growth hormone secretagogue receptor (GHS-R). The GHS-R is expressed in the arcuate nucleus (Arc), along with neuropeptide Y (NPY) neurons. Injections of ghrelin into the arcuate and paraventricular nuclei of the hypothalamus increased food intake in male and female rats (18).

When administered to humans, ghrelin stimulates appetite and food intake, including increased preprandial hunger and meal initiation. Produced by the stomach and duodenum (19), ghrelin increases with fasting and is suppressed with refeeding. Increased ghrelin levels have also been noted in patients with anorexia nervosa and those with Prader-Willi syndrome (20). Ghrelin acts as a stimulator of growth hormone secretion in both animals and humans and has been shown to have a more potent action than that of growth hormone–releasing hormone (21). Ghrelin may also affect energy utilization; it has also been shown in rodents that peripheral daily administration of ghrelin causes weight gain by reducing fat utilization without a significant change in food intake (22).

Satiety

Satiety has been associated with increased activity in the prefrontal cortex (23). This area exerts inhibitory effects on responses to internal and external stimuli. Patients with damage to the prefrontal cortex have hyperphagia (24,25).

The effects of food in the prefrontal cortex have also been found to mimic that of drugs (26). Food is used to self-medicate for distress (27), and sweet foods have been shown to have an analgesic effect (28).

Excessive food intake can induce downregulation, sensitization, and withdrawal and result in choosing the immediate reward of eating even in the face of negative long-term consequences (25).

The prefrontal cortex is involved in the system necessary for decision making and choosing among options for action. In particular, its critical function in this process is to activate feelings or emotional states, which help focus decision making, from "thoughts" about rewarding or punishing events that are not currently present in one's immediate environment (29,30). Davis et al. (25) found that decision-making deficits were greater in women with higher body mass indexes (BMIs) than in normal weight women and suggested that cortical functions that inhibit short-term rewards in the face of long-term negative consequences may be impaired.

A direct and inverse relationship exists between gastric distension and satiety (13). Increasing the food volume but not the energy content of food infused into the stomach has been found to reduce hunger ratings and food intake in both normal weight and obese women (31). Gastrointestinal hormones such as cholecystokinin (CCK) and glucagon-like peptide 1 (GLP-1) can regulate satiety. Sensitivity to the short-term signals produced by CCK and GLP-1 is modulated by leptin, insulin, and ghrelin, which are involved with long-term energy regulation, thereby linking these two systems (32). GLP-1 is a gastrointestinal peptide produced in the ileum in response to ingested carbohydrates and fat. It stimulates the islet cells in the pancreas to secrete insulin and has been shown to reduce appetite and body weight (33).

CCK delays gastric emptying and depends on a distended stomach for effect. CCK signals travel via the vagus nerve, which transmits neuronal signals to the nucleus tractus solitarius and from there to the hypothalamus (34). CCK is released into the blood as a result of the presence of fat or protein in the duodenum. Different types of foods may cause different CCK responses, with foods containing longer chain fatty acids causing a higher release of CCK than those with shorter chain fatty acids (35).

ENERGY UTILIZATION

Regulation of energy utilization is less well understood than that of energy intake. An observational population-based study of children concluded that correlations within groups of spontaneous physical activity suggested the presence of an "activity stat," indicating that activity was centrally and biologically regulated (36).

Spontaneous physical activity, such as fidgeting and time spent moving or standing, may be affected by stimulation of the lateral hypothalamus. Orexins, neuropeptides located in the lateral hypothalamus, may be one link between feeding and spontaneous physical activity (37). In animals, centrally administered orexin increases food intake, waking time, motor activity, and metabolic rate, along with heart rate and blood pressure (38).

ENERGY BALANCE

Energy balance is maintained through a complex relationship between energy stores (adipose tissue), energy intake via feedback from the gastrointestinal tract, and energy utilization, all integrated at the level of the hypothalamus. The complex system regulating energy balance is centered in the hypothalamus (Fig. 3.1).

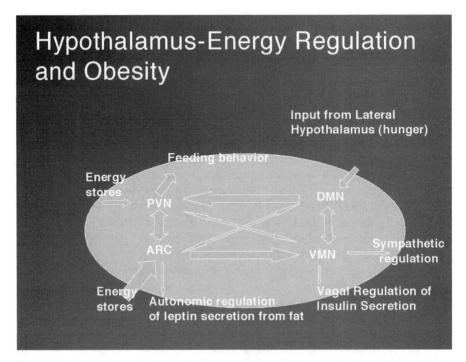

FIG. 3.1. Input to the hypothalamus from energy stores and hunger signals are integrated with efferent output regarding feeding behavior, insulin secretion, and autonomic regulation of adipokines.

Leptin, produced in adipocytes, is correlated to the body's total fat stores. Leptin regulates long-term energy balance in favor of conservation of fat mass (39). Melanocyte–stimulating hormone interacts at the level of the hypothalamus with a melanocortin receptor, MC4-R, to decrease food intake and increase energy expenditure (39). Appetite-stimulating (orexigenic) peptides such as agouti-related protein and neuropeptide Y are also expressed in the hypothalamus as a component of the CNS control of energy balance (39). Gut hormones such as CCK, ghrelin, and peptide YY and vagal nerve signals also input information at the hypothalamic level to regulate hunger and satiety (39).

Adipokines

Adipose tissue itself is a major factor in dynamic energy regulation.

Far from being simply a storage compartment for fat as an energy reserve, the adipose tissue system is an active endocrine organ system. Adipose tissue is composed of brown and white adipose tissue. White adipose tissue is the predominant tissue found in excess in obesity. Brown adipose tissue is present in the newborn and increases in states of cold exposure and starvation. White adipose tissue is made up of an array of cellular types: adipocytes; multipotent stem cells capable of differentiating into muscle, cartilage, adipose tissue, and bone; vascular endothelial cells; stromal cells; and macrophages (Fig. 3.2).

The adipocyte is of particular importance in energy balance. In addition to storing fuel, the adipocyte produces cytokines; participates in hormonal regulation, particularly glucose homeostasis; and is involved in energy regulation/signaling at the level of the CNS and peripheral tissues. A sampling of cytokines produced by the adipocyte is shown in Table 3.2.

Leptin and Energy Regulation

The identification of leptin provided the initial insight into the complex communication between peripheral energy stores and the central nervous system. Leptin is an adipocyte-produced product of the *OB* gene. Leptin administration to leptin-deficient obese mice reduces weight (40,41). Leptin's major site of production is white adipose tissue, but brown adipose tissue, stomach, placenta, mammary gland, ovarian follicles, and fetal organs have also been shown to produce it (42). Leptin

TABLE 3.2. *Some cytokines produced by the adipocyte*

Leptin	Tumor necrosis factor-α	Retinol binding protein
Adiponectin	Interleukin-6	Angiotensinogen
Resistin	Plasminogen activator inhibitor 1	Acylation stimulating protein

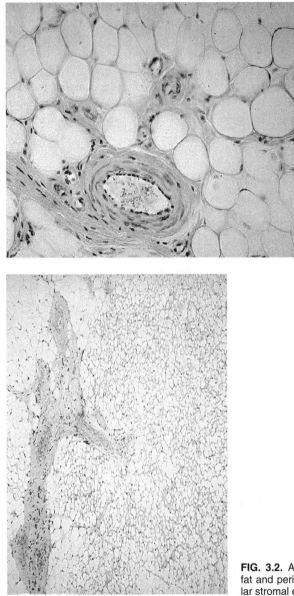

FIG. 3.2. Adipocytes, with centrally stored fat and peripheral nuclei, as well as vascular stromal elements.

receptors have been detected in most tissues, and the hypothalamic nuclei involved in energy regulation are a major target for leptin action.

Leptin also affects expression of the *proopiomelanocortin (POMC)* gene by neurons of the hypothalamic arcuate nucleus (43). As a result α-, β-, and γ-melanocyte–stimulating hormones are produced. These peptides signal target neurons in the lateral hypothalamus that express the melanocortin receptors MC3-R and

MC4-R, which results in decreased food intake and increased energy expenditure (44). Patients with a complete deficiency of POMC due to homozygous or compound heterozygous loss-of-function mutations exhibit a characteristic syndrome marked by childhood-onset severe obesity, red hair, and hypocortisolism (45). The influence of common polymorphisms in POMC, resulting in partial loss of function, on obesity phenotypes in less extreme individuals is unclear (46).

Links to Obesity-Related Comorbidities

Alterations in insulin sensitivity are hallmarks of the metabolic derangements due to obesity and the development of the major comorbidities of type 2 diabetes, dyslipidemia, and cardiovascular disease. Insulin-mediated glucose disposal by muscle varies almost 10-fold in healthy individuals, possibly explaining the variability of the impact of obesity on insulin resistance in each individual. The more insulin sensitive the muscle, the less insulin needs to be secreted to maintain normal glucose homeostasis. The more insulin resistant, the greater the degree of compensatory hyperinsulinemia, and the more likely the individual is to develop disease.

Adipose tissue in obesity becomes refractory to insulin's suppression of fat mobilization, and the resulting insulin resistance increases release of free fatty acids from the adipocytes. Elevated free fatty acid concentrations are linked to the onset of peripheral muscle and hepatic insulin resistance. Hyperinsulinemia stimulates fatty acid synthesis while inhibiting the oxidation of fatty acids and compromising triglyceride transport out of the liver. This results in net accumulation of fat in the hepatocytes and nonalcoholic fatty liver disease (NAFLD). Muscle is also affected; accumulated triacylglycerol inhibits insulin signaling and leads to a reduction in insulin-stimulated muscle glucose transport as well as in muscle glycogen synthesis and glycolysis (47).

Physical activity can decrease insulin resistance even without weight loss. In a study of obese adolescent girls attending a 12-week fitness program, fat-free mass increased, as did insulin sensitivity despite no change in weight or percent body fat (48).

Links between adipokines and cardiovascular disease may arise via adiponectin and its effects on inflammation. A cytokine produced in abundance by adipocytes, adiponectin, varies inversely with adiposity.

Plasma adiponectin concentration is lower in obese individuals than in normal weight persons. Adiponectin is inversely related to insulin levels, inflammatory markers, and fat mass. In adults, reduced adiponectin concentrations have been linked to cardiovascular disease. Physical activity has been found to increase adiponectin levels. In a 3-month physical activity/dietary intervention with adolescents, adiponectin increased by 34%, and fat mass, insulin resistance, and inflammatory factors were reduced despite no significant weight loss (49).

In addition to decreased expression of adiponectin, which has anti-inflammatory action, the secretion of proinflammatory cytokines tumor necrosis factor-α (TNF-α), interleukin-6, prothrombotic factors, and acute phase serum amyloid is increased in obesity (50). These cytokines stimulate macrophage migration into adipose tissue.

Adipocyte-secreted TNF-α stimulates preadipocytes and endothelial cells to produce monocyte chemoattractant protein–1. Increased leptin and decreased adiponectin also stimulate transport of macrophages to adipose tissue, creating a low-grade inflammatory state (51).

A study investigating the effect of lifestyle intervention on inflammatory markers showed an increase in adiponectin, a decrease in C-reactive protein and interleukin (IL)-6, and reduced inflammation in adipose tissue in response to diet and exercise (52). These inflammatory changes may link obesity with cardiovascular disease comorbidity in an as yet unexplained fashion.

CASE

LJ is a 9-year-old African American girl who comes to your office for a "checkup." Her mother and grandmother accompany her. You notice that LJ is tall and looks older than her age. Her weight is 130 lb (>95th percentile), she is 4 ft 11 in. tall (>95th percentile), and her BMI is 26.3 (>95th percentile). Her blood pressure is 115/68 mm Hg. Over the past year, since your last visit with her, she has gained 25 lb. In catching up with the family, you ask how they are doing and the mother notes that she and LJ have moved back in with the grandmother while the mother is going back to school. You ask if they have been concerned about LJ's weight and the mother says she is. The grandmother says that LJ just "likes her food." You review LJ's past history and note that she was a small for dates baby with a maternal history of hypertension and toxemia. Her old growth charts show that although starting out underweight she had rapid "catch-up growth."

LJ's family history is positive for hypertension in the mother and maternal great aunt, for diabetes in the paternal grandfather, and for obesity in the maternal grandmother. Her review of systems yields essentially negative findings.

On physical examination you note that she is Tanner 2 and has mild acanthosis nigricans. You ask about LJ's diet, and the mother says she sometimes skips breakfast, sometimes eats at school. LJ buys lunch at school, and the mother is surprised to find out that the grandmother has been giving LJ extra money for ice cream. After school, the grandmother frequently makes cookies or a special treat for LJ. The family eats dinner together, served family style. Sometimes LJ and her grandmother have a snack together in the evening when watching television. During this review, the mother frequently expresses surprise at the amount LJ is snacking, noting how different this is from the time before they moved back with the grandmother.

It turns out that LJ's level of activity is also low; by the time she finishes her homework, dinner is ready, after which it is dark outside. You calculate with the mother and grandmother that LJ is watching about 4 hours of television per day.

After hearing about LJ's weight gain and your description of her increased risk for heart disease and diabetes, the mother and grandmother decide it is "time to do something." They propose to limit the night-time snacking and let LJ go outdoors after school and finish her homework after dinner. The grandmother also says she will save LJ's school snack money and buy her something special (not food), as well as try to come up with a healthier snack after school.

You order laboratory studies to evaluate LJ's risk for metabolic syndrome, nonalcoholic steatohepatitis (NASH), and dyslipidemia and schedule a return visit for 1 month. One month later, LJ comes back to your office with her grandmother. Her mother is at school but wrote a note saying that the family has been trying hard to work on LJ's weight. In reviewing the results from the laboratory studies you just received, you see that LJ has an increased triglyceride level of 175 mg/dL and a high fasting insulin level of 40 μU/mL, with all other studies within normal limits. You weigh LJ and she has lost 1 lb. The grandmother says the family is "doing well," but about 2 weeks after the last visit, a great aunt passed away and this resulted in more eating away from home and decreased exercise. You encourage the family to continue in their efforts and to complete a diet and activity record. You schedule them to return to your office in 1 month. You ask the grandmother to call and check in with your nurse in 1 to 2 weeks to let you know how they are doing.

On the next visit, you find that LJ has lost 3 lb, she is spending time outdoors every day, and the grandmother has been trying to walk with her about 3 days per week. You review diet records and note the family has been choosing fruit or salad for snacks and LJ has begun to pack her lunch 1 or 2 times per week. You encourage them to continue and arrange to see LJ again in 6 weeks.

REFERENCES

1. Weiss PAM, Scholz HS, Haas J, Tamusinno KF, Seissler J, Borkenstein MH. Long term follow up of infants of mothers with type I diabetes; evidence for hereditary and non hereditary transmission of diabetes and precursors. *Diabetes Care.* 2000;23(7):905–911.
2. Hales CN, Barker DJ, Clark PM, Cox LJ, Fall C, Osmond C, Winter PD . Fetal and infant growth and impaired glucose tolerance at age 64. *BMJ.* 1991;30:1019–1022.
3. Law CM, Barker DJ, Osmond C, Fall CH, Simmonds SJ . Early growth and abdominal fatness in adult life. *J Epidemiol Community Health.* 1992;46(3):184–186.
4. McMillen IC, Robinson JS. Developmental origins of the metabolic syndrome: predication, plasticity, programming. *Physiol Rev.* 2005;85(2):571–633.
5. Toschke AM, Montgomery SM, Pfeiffer U, von Kries R. Early intrauterine exposure to tobacco-inhaled products and obesity. *Am J Epidemiol.* 2003;158:1068–1074.
6. Godfrey KM, Robinson JS, Barker DJ, et al. Maternal nutrition in early and late pregnancy in relation to placental and fetal growth. *Bone Miner J.* 1996;312:410–414.
7. Barker DJ. The intrauterine origins of cardiovascular disease. *Acta Paediatr.* 1993;82(Suppl 391):93–99.
8. Lucas A. Programming by early nutrition in man. *Ciba Found Symp.* 1991;156:38–50.
9. Hay WW. Recent observations on the regulation of fetal metabolism by glucose. *J Physiol.* 2006;572(Pt 1):17–24.
10. Bateson P, Barker D, Clutton-Brock T, Deb D, D'Udine B, Foley RA, Gluckman P, Godfrey K, Kirkwood T, Lahr MM, McNamara J, Metcalfe NB, Monaghan P, Spencer HG, Sultan SE. Developmental plasticity and human health. *Nature.* 2004;430:419–422.
11. Hales CN, Barker DJ. The thrifty phenotype hypothesis. *Br Med Bull.* 2001;60:5–20.
12. Whitaker RC, Wright JA, Pepe MS, Seidel KD, Dietz WH. Predicting obesity in young adulthood from childhood and parental obesity. *N Engl J Med.* 1997;337:869–873.
13. de Graaf C, Blom WA Smeets PA, stafleu A, Hendriks HF. Biomarkers of satiation and satiety. *Am J Clin Nutr.* 2004;79:946–961.
14. Blundell JE, Lawton CL, Cotton JR, Macdiamid JI. Control of human appetite: implications for the intake of dietary fat. *Annu Rev Nutr.* 1996;16:285–319.
15. de Graaf C, DeJong LS, Lambers AC. Palatability affects satiation but not satiety. *Physiol Behav.* 1999;66(4):681–688.
16. Tordorff MG. Obesity by choice the powerful influence of nutrient availability on nutrient intake. *Am J Physiol Regul Integr Comp Physiol.* 2002;282:R1536–1539.

17. O'Dorherty J, Rolls ET, Francis S, Bowtell R, McGlone F. Representation of pleasant and aversive tastes in the human brain. *J Neurophysiol.* 2001;85:1315–1321.
18. Currie PJ, Mirza A, Fuld R, Park D, Vasselli JR. Ghrelin is an anorexigenic and metabolic signaling peptide in the arcuate and paraventricular nucleus. *Am J Physiol Regul Integr Comp Physiol.* 2005;289:R353–358.
19. Kojima M, Hosoda H, Date Y, Nakazato M, Matsuo H, Kangawa K. Ghrelin is a growth-hormone-releasing acylated peptide from stomach. *Nature.* 1999;402:656–660.
20. Cummings DE, Clement K, Purnell JQ, Vaisse C, Foster KE, Frayo RS, Schwartz MW, Basdevant A, Weigle DS. Elevated plasma ghrelin levels in Prader Willi syndrome. *Nat Med.* 2002;8:643–644.
21. Ariyasu H, Takaya K, Tagami T, Ogawa Y, Hosoda K, Akamizu T, Suda M, Koh T, Natsui K, Toyooka S, Shirakami G, Usui T, Shimatsu A, Doi K, Hosoda H, Kojima M, Kangawa K, Nakao K. Stomach is a major source of circulating ghrelin, and feeding state determines plasma ghrelin-like immunoreactivity levels in humans. *J Clin Endocrinol Metab.* 2001;86:4753–4758.
22. Tschöp M, Smiley DL, Heiman ML. Ghrelin induces adiposity in rodents. *Nature.* 2000;407:908–913.
23. Tataranni PA, Gautier JF, Chen K, Uecker A, Bandy D, Salbe AD, Pratley RD, Lawson M, Reimen EM, Ravssun E. Neuroanatomic correlates of hunger and satiation in humans using positron emission tomography. *Proc Natl Acad Sci U S A.* 1999;9:4569–4574.
24. Graff-Radford NR, Russell JW, Rezai K. Frontal degenerative dementia and neuroimaging. *Adv Neurol.* 1995;66:37–47.
25. Davis C, Levitan RD, Muglia P, Bewell C, Kennedy JL. Decision-making deficits and overeating; a risk model for obesity. *Obes Res.* 2004;12:929–935.
26. Schroeder BE, Binzak JM, Kelley AE. A common profile of prefrontal cortical activation following exposure to nicotine- or chocolate-associated contextual cues. *Neuroscience.* 2001;105:535–545.
27. Wallis DJ, Hetherington MM. Stress and eating; the effects of ego-threat and cognitive demand on food intake in restrained and emotional eaters. *Appetite.* 2004;4391:39–46.
28. Mercer ME, Holder MD. Antinociceptive effects of palatable sweet ingesta on human responsivity to pressure pain. *Physiol Behav.* 1997;61:311–318.
29. Bechara A, Damasio H, Damasio AR, Lee GP. Different contributions of the human amygdala and ventromedial prefrontal cortex to decision-making. *J Neurosci.* 1999;19:5473–5481.
30. Bechara A, Damasio AR, Damasio H. Emotion, decision-making, and the orbitofrontal cortex. *Cereb Cortex.* 2000;10:295–307.
31. Rolls BJ, Roe LS. Effect of the volume of liquid food infused intragastrically on satiety in women. *Physiol Behav.* 2002;76(4-5):623–631.
32. Havel PJ. Peripheral signals conveying metabolic information to the brain: short term and long term regulation of food intake and energy homeostasis. *Exp Biol Med (Maywood).* 2001;226(11):963–977.
33. Zander M, Madsbad S, Madson JL, Holst JJ. Effect of 6 week course of glucagon like peptide 1 on glycemic control, insulin sensitivity, and beta cell function in type 2 diabetes: a parallel group study. *Lancet.* 2002;359:824–830.
34. Kisseleff HR, Carretta JC, Geleibter A, Pi Sunyer FX. Cholecystokinin and stomach distension combine to reduce food intake in humans. *Am J Physiol Regul Integr Comp Physiol.* 2003;285:R992–998.
35. Matzinger D, Degen L, Drewe J, Meuli J, Duebendorfer R, Ruckstuhl N, D'Amato M, Rovati L, Berlinger C. The role of long chain fatty acids in regulating food intake and cholecystokinin release in humans. *Gut.* 2000;46:688–693.
36. Wilkin TJ, Mallam KM, Metcalf BS, Jeffery AN, Voss LD. Variation in physical activity lies with the child, not his environment: evidence for an 'activitystat' in young children (EarlyBird 16). *Int J Obes. (Lond)* 2006;30(7):1050–1055.
37. Kotz CM. Integration of feeding and spontaneous physical activity: role for orexin. *Physiol Behav.* 2006;88(3):294–301.
38. Sakurai T. Orexin: a link between energy homeostasis and adaptive behaviour. *Curr Opin Clin Nutr Metab Care.* 2003;6940:353–360.
39. Korner J, Leibel RL. To eat or not to eat—how the gut talks to the brain. *N Engl J Med.* 2003;349:926–927.
40. Maffei M, Fei H, Lee GH, Dani C, Leroy P, Zahang Y, Proenca R, Negrel R, Aihaud G, Friedman JM. Increased expression in adipocytes of ob RNA in mice with lesions of the hypothalamus and with mutations at the db locus. *Proc Natl Acad Sci U S A.* 1995;92(15):6957–6960.
41. Halaas JL, Gajiwala KS, Maffei M, Cohen SL, Chait BT, Rabinowitz D, Lallone RL, Burley SK, Friedman JM. Weight-reducing effects of the plasma protein encoded by the obese gene. *Science.* 1995;269:543–546.

42. Green ED, Maffei M, Braden VV, Proenca R, DeSilva U, Zhang Y, Chua SC, Leibel RL, Weissenbach J, Friedman JM. The human obese (OB) gene: RNA expression pattern and mapping on the physical, cytogenetic and genetic maps of chromosome 7. *Genome Res.* 1995;5(1):5–12.
43. Baker M, Gaukrodger N, Mayosi BM, Imrie H, Farrall M, Watkins H, Connell JM, Avery PJ, Keavney B. Association between common polymorphisms of the proopiomelanocortin gene and body fat distribution: a family study. *Diabetes.* 2005;54:2492–2499.
44. Yeo GS, Farooqi IS, Challis BG, Jackson RS, O'Rahilly S . The role of melanocortin signaling in the control of body weight: evidence from human and murine genetic models. *Q J Med.* 2000;9391: 7–14.
45. Krude H, Biebermann H, Luck W, Horn R, Brabant G, Gruters A. Severe early-onset obesity, adrenal insufficiency and red hair pigmentation caused by POMC mutations in humans. *Nat Genet.* 1998;19:155–157.
46. Krude H, Biebermann H, Gruters A. Mutations in the human proopiomelanocortin gene. *Ann N Y Acad Sci.* 2003;994:233–239.
47. Kovacs P, Stumvoll M. Fatty acids and insulin resistance in muscle and liver. *Best Pract Res Clin Endocrinol Metab.* 2005;19:625–635.
48. Nassis GP, Papantakou K, Skenderi K, Triandafillopoulou M, Kavouras SA, Yannakoulia M, Chrousos GP, Sidossis LS. Aerobic exercise training improves insulin sensitivity without changes in body weight, body fat, adiponectin, and inflammatory markers in overweight and obese girls. *Metabolism.* 2005;54:1472–1479.
49. Balagopal P, George D, Yarandi H, Funanage V, Bayne E. Reversal of obesity related hypoadiponectinemia by lifestyle intervention: a controlled, randomized study in obese adolescents. *J Clin Endocrinol Metab.* 2005;90:6192–6197.
50. Yang RZ, Lee MJ, Hu H, Pollin TI, Ryan AS, Nicklas BJ, Snitker S, Horenstein RB, Hull K, Goldberg NH, Goldberg AP, Shuldiner AR, Fried SK, Gong DW. Acute phase serum amyloid A: an inflammatory adipokine and potential link between obesity and its metabolic complications. *PLoS Med.* 2006;3(6):e287.
51. Wellen KI, Hotamisligil GS. Obesity-induced inflammatory changes in adipose tissue. *J Clin Invest.* 2003;112:1785–1788.
52. Bruun JM, Helge JW, Richelsen B, Stallknecht B. Diet and exercise reduce low grade inflammation and macrophage infiltration in adipose tissue but not in skeletal muscle in severely obese subjects. *Am J Physiol Endocrinol Metab.* 2006;290:E961–967.

4

Obesity in the Context of Child and Adolescent Development

Obesity results from energy imbalance and is the final common pathway of deviations from the individual's optimal energy intake and expenditure. Children, in contrast to adults, have a requirement for growth that operates in addition to all the other modifiers of energy balance (Table 4.1). There may be critical periods of development in childhood that are especially sensitive to obesity-promoting factors and increase the likelihood of later obesity. The intrauterine environment has been found to have a much greater impact on later obesity and obesity-related comorbidities than previously thought. Feeding patterns and breastfeeding or formula feeding have a lasting influence on obesity risk and susceptibility. Rapid weight gain in early childhood, causing a crossing of growth percentiles (adiposity rebound), may predict obesity later in life. Emotional and psychological factors in the child or adolescent and parenting style and interaction can have an impact beyond childhood. Shared family environment and learned behavior can magnify a child's predisposition for obesity. Awareness of this complex interplay of influences affecting an obese child or adolescent can help in developing a strategy for regaining energy balance (Fig 4.1). Individual child, family, and community factors can affect energy intake and expenditure (Fig 4.2).

INTRAUTERINE INFLUENCES AND OBESITY

Influences on energy regulation begin during intrauterine life, and the intrauterine environment is thought to have a significant effect on later obesity. Infants born to diabetic mothers tend to have a greater amount of adipose tissue and an increased

TABLE 4.1. *Factors affecting energy balance in children and adolescents*

• Genetic predisposition	• Family influences
• Requirements for growth	• Activity opportunities
• Interactions with the nutritional environment	• Motor development
	• Emotional/psychological states

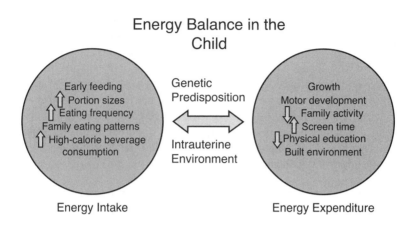

FIG. 4.1. Factors influencing energy balance in the child.

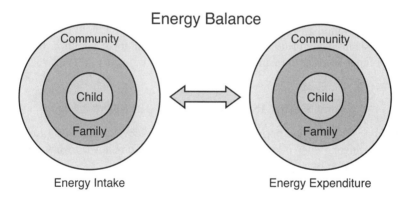

FIG. 4.2. Energy balance in the context of the child.

likelihood of developing obesity, impaired glucose tolerance, and type 2 diabetes during childhood (1). The effects of the intrauterine environment may persist over time. Children whose mothers were diabetic during pregnancy had greater rates of obesity at the ages of 5 to 9 years than expected in a normal population (2). Nine- to 14-year-old children of mothers with gestational diabetes had greater rates of obesity independent of physical activity, television watching, energy intake, breastfeeding duration, mother's body mass index (BMI), and other maternal and family variables than children born to mothers without diabetes during pregnancy (3).

Exposure to excess of glucose and resulting hyperinsulinemia *in utero* may alter insulin receptor expression and insulin sensitivity to the extrauterine environment (4).

As the obesity epidemic worsens and the prevalence of diabetes in adult and young adult women increases, the risk of pregnancy complicated by diabetes will increase as well. This will mean that infants from these pregnancies will have greater risk for future obesity and diabetes, and a vicious cycle of increasing obesity and obesity-related comorbidity will be created. Unexpectedly, infants born small for gestational age have also been found to have an increased incidence of obesity in childhood (5), particularly if they are introduced into an energy-rich environment, which causes rapid growth. Intrauterine growth in a restrictive nutritional environment due to maternal undernutrition may lead to exposure to increased amounts of fatty acids, which can stimulate adipose tissue hyperplasia (6). External factors such as maternal hypertension and smoking can increase the risk for reduced intrauterine growth and become additive risk factors for obesity.

Infants born of a diabetic pregnancy, small for gestational age infants who have experienced rapid catch-up growth, and infants in families in which a parent or parents are obese are all at risk for childhood obesity.

In addition to optimizing nutrition and activity habits for all children and families, these at-risk infants and their families may need additional attention focused on energy balance in order to maintain a normal growth trajectory.

EARLY INFLUENCES ON OBESITY

The first year of life is a period of rapid growth and development. And early nutrition can influence later obesity. Breastfeeding has been shown to have a role in reducing later obesity.

Proposed mechanisms include effects on total caloric intake, insulin secretion, and modulation of fat deposition (7). Rate of weight gain between birth and 4 months of age as well as birth weight has been associated with an increased risk of obesity at age 7 years (8) and at age 20 years (9). Rates of weight gain vary greatly in the first 1 to 2 years of life, with growth in infants accelerating or decelerating across percentiles (10). Infants who showed growth accelerations in weight between birth and age 2 years have been found to be heavier and taller, with a greater percentage of body fat, at age 5 years. Children who were lighter, shorter, and thinner at birth (signs of intrauterine growth restraint) were more likely to experience "catch-up" weight gain (10). The mechanism for this catch-up growth is not known, although greater food intake has been observed (10). Leptin has been proposed as a possible mediator of this effect. Concentrations of cord blood leptin are positively correlated with birth weight but inversely related to weight gain in infancy; low concentrations at birth may induce catch-up growth by reducing inhibition of satiety (11). There is evidence that early adiposity rebound is a predictor of childhood, adolescent, and adult obesity. Adiposity rebound is the rise in BMI after reaching a nadir in the child at 4 to 6 years of age (12). Another way of viewing adiposity rebound is as a descriptor of the phenomenon of "crossing growth percentiles."

Parent factors and parent-child interactions can affect weight gain in a child. In a prospective study of children from birth to 9.5 years of age, five independent risk factors for childhood overweight were found. *Parental overweight* was the strongest factor, which was mediated by the *child's temperament.* The remaining risk factors were *low parental concerns about the child's thinness,* the *child's persistent tantrums over food,* and *less sleep time in childhood* (13).

Attention to detail is important because small energy imbalances in feeding and eating patterns, activity patterns, and parent-child interactions around food can result, over time, in significant weight gain. For example, if a child either consumes 150 kcal/day or reduces activity expenditure by 150 kcal/day, he or she will gain 15 lb over the course of 1 year (Fig. 4.3).

EMOTIONAL AND PSYCHOLOGICAL STRESS

Psychological and emotional states have often been linked to changes in weight. In one study, oppositional defiant disorder was found more commonly in children who were chronically obese during childhood and adolescence than in normal weight children or children who either developed obesity in childhood and then normalized their weight or developed obesity in adolescence. Among this same group of chronically obese children, boys had higher rates of depression than did children in other weight categories (14).

Depression has been found to predict obesity. In a study of adolescents in 7th to 12th grade, those who had a depressed mood were more likely to have follow-up obesity. In contrast, obesity at the start of the study did not predict follow-up depression (15).

FAMILY INFLUENCE ON ENERGY BALANCE

Nutritional Influences

Parents and families clearly influence the nutritional environment of their children. These influences can be subtle. In a study of 3- to 5-year-olds over a 6-year period, children's body fat increased linearly with parent disinhibition. Parental dietary restraint was also associated with the child's increase in body fat when coupled with disinhibition. The authors speculated that this association could be "mediated by direct parental role modeling of unhealthy eating behaviors, or through other indirect, and probably subconscious, behavioral consequences such as the suppression of the child's innate regulation of dietary intake" (16). In addition to directly affecting eating behavior and modeling, and healthy eating habits, parents play a major role in determining the child's and family's nutritional environment and negotiating lifestyle change.

Parental involvement is essential in obesity intervention.

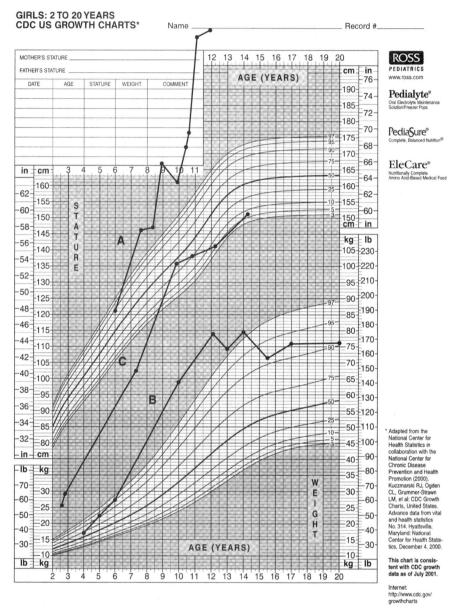

FIG. 4.3. In this example, *curve B* represents an excess weight gain of 7.5 lb/year between the ages of 6 and 12 years. This represents a daily calorie excess of 75 kcal. *Curve C* illustrates the impact of early weight gain. Patient C weighed 55 lb at age 2 years. From age 2 to 6 years she gained 18 lb/year, representing an excess calorie imbalance of 16 lb/year, or 160 kcal/day. *Curve A* represents an excess weight gain over the 6 years between the ages of 6 and 12 years of 19 lb/year, or 190 kcal/day.

Children of parents who took charge of the lifestyle changes in the family lost more weight than did children in families in which the child was the person responsible for the change (17). This study also supported an authoritative parenting style, which is defined as firm and supportive parenting. Parents were encouraged to assume a leadership role in the environmental change, allowing for appropriate granting of a child's autonomy in modifying family and child nutrition and activity (18). Parenting skills that target gradual increases in activity and reduction in high-fat, high-calorie foods are considered essential in obesity treatment (19).

ACTIVITY OPPORTUNITIES

Energy expenditure is the other modifiable component of the energy equation. Energy expenditure in childhood and adolescence varies with developmental stage; opportunities in the community for physical activity; and family, school, and peer influences.

Obesity itself can impact the ability to exercise.

On exercise testing, morbidly obese adolescents were found to have severe deconditioning (20) with exercise capability far below that of normal weight peers. In another study, obese adolescents performed significantly more poorly on walk-run and unloaded cycling testing, which was thought to be due to increased energy demands required to move excess body weight (21).

In a group of prepubertal children, similar findings showed that walking and running were energetically more costly for obese children, based on their excess weight. Calorie expenditure was comparable in the obese and normal weight groups when calculated by energy expenditure per body weight or fat-free mass (22). In a study of prepubertal children, total energy expenditure was correlated with body weight, fat-free mass, resting energy expenditure, and peak VO_2 max during exercise. Reduced energy expenditure has been found in a group of infants prior to the development of obesity (23). However, other studies have not identified a link between total energy expenditure and subsequent obesity (24). Although there is no clear evidence that explains the link between total energy expenditure and the etiology of obesity, there is evidence that the quality and duration of physical activity can be a factor in maintaining energy balance (25).

Obese children and adolescents may face barriers to increasing activity.

Overweight girls report more body-related resource and social barriers to physical activity than normal weight girls, with overweight boys reporting higher body-related barriers than normal weight boys. Body-related barriers are related to self-consciousness about looks when engaging in physical activity. Resource issues

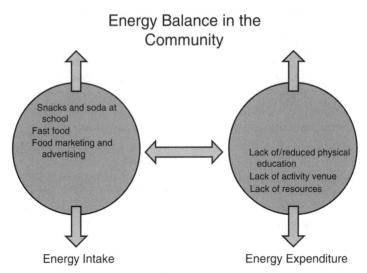

FIG. 4.4. Energy imbalance in the community.

include lack of skills, equipment, knowledge, and interest as well as a place to do physical activity. Lack of partners for physical activities and teasing constitute social barriers to physical activity (26). Families need to be aware of these factors in order to facilitate an increase in their obese child's or adolescent's activity.

> Television, video games, and computers all contribute to increased sedentary activity.

A study showed that children who watched television at least 4 hours per day were less likely to engage in vigorous physical activity and had greater BMIs and skin fold measurements than those who watched television less than 2 hours per day (27). A randomized controlled study, which resulted in reduced television viewing in first-grade children, led to significant relative decreases in BMI (28). Maternal depression has been linked to increased television watching in children and was found to be additive to maternal obesity as a risk factor for this behavior (29). Parents clearly have a role in limiting television viewing and screen time and need to be aware that in so doing they are making a major contribution to their child's health.

INFLUENCE OF THE COMMUNITY

Community factors can also affect energy balance in terms of available activity environments, maximizing physical activity and nutrition in schools, and attention to healthy eating environments and marketing strategies (Fig. 4.4).

REFERENCES

1. Dabelea D, Pettitt DJ. Intrauterine diabetic environment confers risks for type 2 diabetes mellitus and obesity in the offspring in addition to genetic susceptibility. *J Pediatr Endocrinol Metab.* 2001;14: 1085–1091.
2. Plagemann A, Harder T, Kohlhoff R, Rohde W, Dorner G. Overweight and obesity in infants of mothers with long-term insulin dependent diabetes or gestational diabetes. *Int J Obes Relat Metab Disord.* 1997;21:451–456.
3. Gillman MW, Rifas-Shiman S, Berkey CS, Field AE, Colditz GA. Maternal gestational diabetes, birth weight and adolescent obesity. *Pediatrics.* 2003;111(3):e221–e226.
4. Freinkel N. Of pregnancy and progeny (Banting lecture 1980). *Diabetes.* 1980;29:1023–1035.
5. Veening M, Van Weissenbruch M, Delemarre-Van de Wall H. Glucose tolerance, insulin sensitivity and insulin secretion in children born small for gestational age. *J Clin Endocrinol Metab.* 2001; 879:4657–4661.
6. Martin RJ, Hausman GJ, Hausman DB. Regulation of adipose cell development in utero. *Proc Soc Exp Biol Med.* 1998;219:200–210.
7. Owen CG, Martin RM, Whinecup PH Smith GD, Cook DG. Effect of infant feeding on the risk of obesity across the life course: a quantitative review of published evidence. *Pediatrics.* 2005;115: 1367–1377.
8. Stettler N, Zernel BS, Kumanyika S, Stallings VA. Infant weight gain and childhood overweight status in a multicenter cohort study. *Pediatrics.* 2002;109:192–199.
9. Stettler N, Kumanyika SK, Katz SH, Zernel BS, Stallings VA. Rapid weight gain during infancy and obesity in young adulthood in a cohort of African Americans. *Am J Clin Nutr.* 2003;77:1374–1378.
10. Ong KK, Ahmed ML, Emmett PM, Preece MA, Dunger DB. Association between postnatal catch-up growth and obesity in childhood: prospective cohort study. *BMJ.* 2000;320:967–971.
11. Ong KK, Ahmed ML, Sherriff A, Woods KA, Watts A, Golding J, Dunger DB. Cord blood leptin is associated with size at birth and predicts infancy weight gain in humans ALSPAC Study Team. Avon Longitudinal Study of Pregnancy and Childhood. *J Clin Endocrinol Metab.* 1999;84:1145–1148.
12. Whitaker RC, Pepe MS, Wright JA, Seidel KD, Dietz WH. Early adiposity rebound and the risk of adult obesity. *Pediatrics.* 1998;101:E5.
13. Agras WS, Hammer LD, McNicholas F, Kraemer HC. Risk factors for childhood overweight: a prospective study from birth to 9.5 years. *J Pediatr.* 2004;15:20–25.
14. Mustillo S, Worthman C, Erkanli A, Keeler G, Angold A, Costello EJ. Obesity and psychiatric disorder: developmental trajectories. *Pediatrics.* 2003;111(4 Pt 1):851–859.
15. Goodman E, Whitaker RC. A prospective study of the role of depression in the development and persistence of adolescent obesity. *Pediatrics.* 2002;110:497–504.
16. Hood MY, Moore LL, Sundarajan-Ramamurti A, Singer M, Cupplies LA, Ellison RC. Parental eating attitudes and the development of obesity in children. The Framingham Children's Study. *Int J Obes Relat Metab Disord.* 2000;24:1319–1325.
17. Golan M, Weizman A, Apter A, Fainaru M. Parents as exclusive agents of change in the treatment of childhood obesity. *Am J Clin Nutr.* 1998;67:1130–1135.
18. Golan M, Crow S. Targeting parents exclusively in the treatment of childhood obesity: long term results. *Obes Res.* 2004;12:357–361.
19. Barlow SE, Dietz WH. Obesity evaluation and treatment: Expert Committee recommendations. The Maternal and Child Health Bureau, Health Resources and Services Administration and the Department of Health and Human Services. *Pediatrics.* 1998;102:E29.
20. Gidding SS, Nehgme R, Heise C, Hassink S. Severe obesity associated with cardiovascular deconditioning, high prevalence of cardiovascular risk factors, diabetes mellitus/hyperinsulinemia, and respiratory compromise. *J Pediatr.* 2004;144:766–769.
21. Norman AC, Drinkard B, McDuffie JR, Ghorbani S, Yanoff LB, Yanovski, JA. Influence of excess adiposity on exercise fitness and performance in overweight children and adolescents. *Pediatrics.* 2005;115:e690–e696.
22. Maffeis C, Schutz Y, Schena F, Zaffanello M, Pinelli L. Energy expenditure during walking and running in obese and nonobese prepubertal children. *J Pediatr.* 1993;123:193–199.
23. Roberts SB, Savage J, Coward WA, Chew B, Lucas A. Energy expenditure and intake in infants born to lean and overweight mothers. *N Engl J Med.* 1988;318:461–466.
24. Stunkard AJ, Berkowitz RI, Stalling VA, Scholeller DA. Energy intake, not energy output, is a determinant of body size in infants. *Am J Clin Nutr.* 1999;69:524–530.

25. Goran ML, Sun M. Total energy expenditure and physical activity in prepubertal children; recent advances based on doubly labeled water method. *Am J Clin Nutr.* 1998;68:944S–999S.
26. Zabinkski M, Saelens BE, Stein RI, Hayden-Wade HA, Wilfley DE. Overweight children's barriers to and support for physical activity. *Obes Res.* 2003;11:238–246.
27. Anderson RE, Crespo CJ, Bartlett SJ, Cheskin LJ, Pratt M. Relationship of physical activity and television watching with body weight and level of fatness among children: results from the Third National Health and Nutrition Examination Survey. *JAMA.* 1998;279:938–942.
28. Robinson TN. Reducing children's television viewing to prevent obesity. A randomized controlled trial. *JAMA.* 1999;282:1561–1567.
29. Burdette HL, Whitaker RC, Kahn RS, Harvey-Berino J. Association of maternal obesity and depressive symptoms with television-viewing time in low-income preschool children. *Arch Pediatr Adolesc Med.* 2003;157:894–899.

5

Evaluation of the Obese Child

GROWTH

The first step in the evaluation of the obese child or adolescent is determining the height and weight and calculating the body mass index (BMI) (1). Data for the current BMI curves represent cross-sectional data from the U.S. population collected between 1963 and 1980. BMI is highly correlated with increased adiposity in children and adolescents with BMI greater than the 85th percentile for age and gender (2).

The Centers for Disease Control and Prevention (CDC) considers children and adolescents whose BMI is between the 85th and 95th percentiles to be "at risk for overweight," and children and adolescents with a BMI greater than the 95th percentile are considered to be "overweight" (1). There is growing consensus for using the term *obesity* to describe children whose BMI is greater than the 95th percentile and *overweight* to describe children whose BMI is between the 85th and 95th percentiles (3) to more clearly indicate the risk of having a BMI greater than the 95th percentile in terms of obesity-related comorbidities.

BMI is calculated as weight (kg) / height (m^2) or weight (lb) / height (in.^{2}) $\times$ 703. The result is plotted against age on a gender-specific BMI curve (Figs. 5.1 and 5.2).

BMI will help identify children who are obese (BMI >95th percentile), overweight (BMI between the 85th and 95th percentiles), normal weight (BMI between the 5th and 85th percentiles), or underweight (BMI <5th percentile for age and gender). When applied to an individual child, the calculation of BMI allows for classification and prompts further evaluation of individual risk factors for obesity and obesity-related comorbidities. If a child is younger than 2 years, then length-for-height measurements are plotted (Figs. 5.3 and 5.4).

Patterns of weight and BMI change can also be very informative. Children or adolescents who are crossing percentiles are at risk for continued weight gain (1), and a thorough evaluation of activity, inactivity, and nutritional habits would be indicated.

CDC Growth Charts: United States

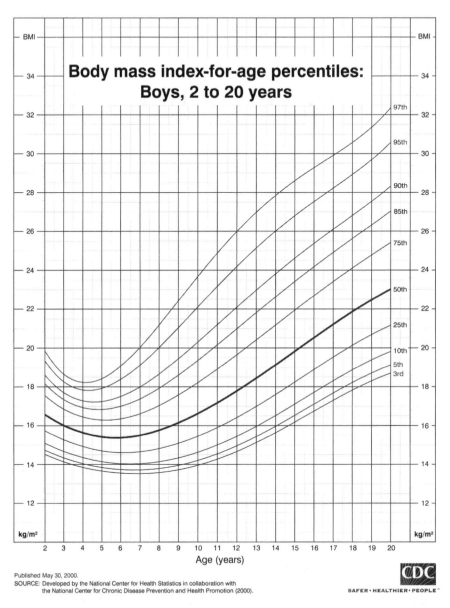

FIG. 5.1. Body mass index-for-age percentiles: boys 2 to 20 years. (Developed by the National Center for Health Statistics in collaboration with the National Center for Chronic Disease.)

CDC Growth Charts: United States

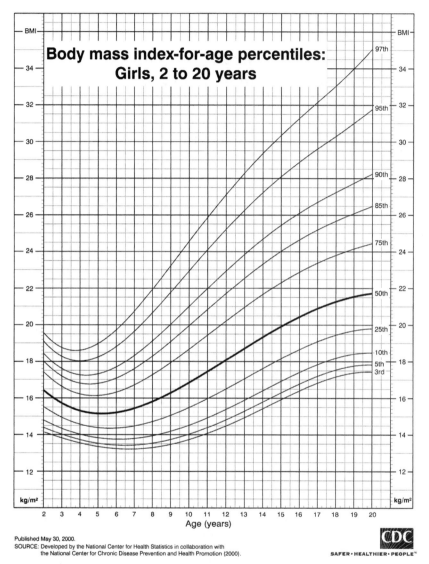

Body mass index-for-age percentiles: Girls, 2 to 20 years

Age (years)

Published May 30, 2000.
SOURCE: Developed by the National Center for Health Statistics in collaboration with
the National Center for Chronic Disease Prevention and Health Promotion (2000).

SAFER·HEALTHIER·PEOPLE™

FIG. 5.2. Body mass index-for-age percentiles: girls 2 to 20 years. (Developed by the National Center for Health Statistics in collaboration with the National Center for Chronic Disease.)

CDC Growth Charts: United States

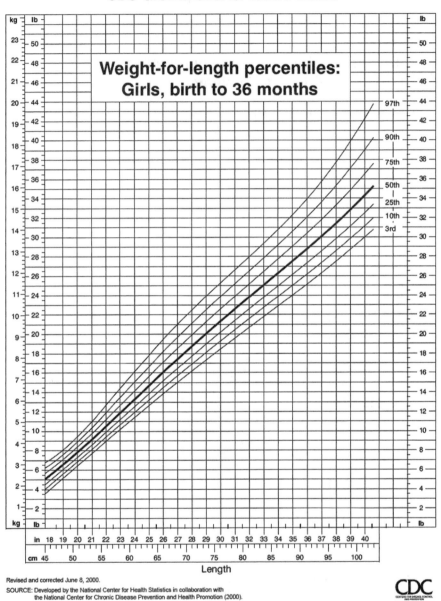

Weight-for-length percentiles:
Girls, birth to 36 months

Revised and corrected June 8, 2000.

SOURCE: Developed by the National Center for Health Statistics in collaboration with
the National Center for Chronic Disease Prevention and Health Promotion (2000).

CDC

FIG: 5.3. Weight-for-length percentiles: girls birth to 36 months. (Developed by the National Center for Health Statistics in collaboration with the National Center for Chronic Disease.)

CDC Growth Charts: United States

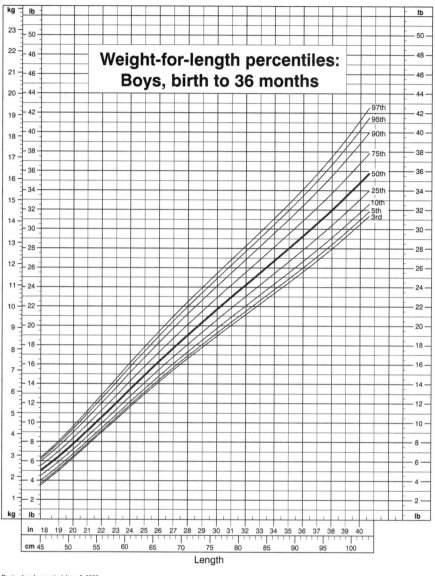

Weight-for-length percentiles:
Boys, birth to 36 months

Length

Revised and corrected June 5, 2000.
SOURCE: Developed by the National Center for Health Statistics in collaboration with
    the National Center for Chronic Disease Prevention and Health Promotion (2000).

FIG. 5.4. Weight-for-length percentiles: boys birth to 36 months. (Developed by the National Center for Health Statistics in collaboration with the National Center for Chronic Disease.)

In addition, weight gain may often accompany stressful situations in a young person's life, such as the following:

- Parental divorce
- Family illness
- Difficult school change
- Onset of depression (4)

Examining the child's situation at the time weight gain occurred may give direction to the kind of intervention required to regain energy balance.

Once a child is found to have a BMI greater than the 95th percentile, the physician must screen for obesity-related risk of disease. Then the child's or adolescent's nutrition, activity, and inactivity patterns should be assessed to determine the potential for change as it involves the child, the family, and the environment. Families should be engaged in a dialogue about value for change, prioritization of needed changes, and strategies for family-based change to begin helping the child achieve a healthier weight (1).

ASSESSMENT OF OBESITY-RELATED COMORBIDITIES

The remainder of this book addresses obesity-related comorbidities in detail. Table 5.1 presents those comorbidities that need to be assessed when the clinician has determined that a child is overweight or obese.

Laboratory Testing

Fasting glucose, insulin, lipid profile, and liver enzyme tests have been recommended in children with a BMI greater than the 95th percentile (1). Other laboratory

TABLE 5.1. *Obesity-related comorbidities*

Central nervous system (CNS)	Orthopedic
Pseudotumor cerebri	Blount's disease
Hypothalamic obesity	Slipped capital femoral epiphysis
Respiratory	Endocrine
Asthma	Metabolic syndrome
Sleep apnea	Impaired glucose tolerance
Obesity hypoventilation syndrome	Diabetes
Cardiovascular	Cushing's disease
Hypertension	Hypothyroidism
Left ventricular hypertrophy	Polycystic ovarian syndrome
Dyslipidemia	Genetic
Gastrointestinal	Prader-Willi syndrome
Nonalcoholic steatohepatitis	Bardet-Biedl syndrome
Cholelithiasis	Alstrom's syndrome
Gastroesophageal reflux	Psychological (other)
Renal	Depression
Glomerulosclerosis	Anxiety
	Low self-esteem
	Binge eating disorder

testing is based on clinical evaluation, family history, and signs and/or symptoms of comorbid conditions.

Assessment and Treatment of Energy Imbalance

> Obesity is an excess of adipose tissue, created and maintained by an ongoing mismatch between energy intake and energy utilization.

In addition to determining the growth pattern of height, weight, and BMI over time, it is important to identify the sources of the energy imbalance and the possible areas where this imbalance can be corrected. To do so, energy intake and energy output need to be assessed, as well as factors that may encourage or impede lifestyle changes that need to occur. Numerous guidelines suggesting a balanced approach to preventing and treating obesity have been published (1,5–7).

Nutritional Assessment

In the nutritional assessment, imbalance of nutrients, portion size, sugar-sweetened beverages, fast food, and frequent snacking are common findings in the diets of overweight youngsters.

> A detailed dietary history is essential.

Asking the child to begin in the morning and go through his or her day will give the pediatrician a good working idea of nutritional factors that are in need of change. For example, a typical 1-day dietary history for an obese adolescent might show that breakfast was skipped, lunch was a soft pretzel and juice, and the after school snack consisted of a bag of chips and soda purchased at the local store. Dinner might be pizza eaten out with the family, and snack food with soda might comprise the nighttime eating. At this point, more than enough information has been given to begin the process of change.

Consumption of sugar-sweetened beverages has been linked to obesity (8). In a prospective study that eliminated sugar-sweetened beverages, adolescents in the upper one third of the BMI range had significant decreases in BMI compared with similar adolescents who drank sugar-sweetened beverages (9).

One of the potential contributors to energy imbalance has been the increase in portion size (10). If children are offered larger portions, they will eat more food (11). Consumption of fast food is another factor in increasing energy imbalance. A large household survey revealed that one third of children eat fast food every day. Consumption of fast food was associated with a caloric increase of 187 kcal/day and a diet that included greater amounts of fat, carbohydrate, sugar, and sugar-sweetened beverages and reduced intake of fiber, fruits, and vegetables (12). Increasing fruit, vegetable (13), and dairy consumption (14) has been associated with improved energy balance.

It is always important to identify the nutritional environments the child is exposed to during the day or week. Parents may not know what meals and snacks day care may be providing, and need to be encouraged to ask for menus. Many schools are trying to improve the nutritional quality of their breakfast and lunch programs; however, the meals in some schools are still problematic and a packed lunch would be an improvement. By the same token, vending machines may be filled with soda and unhealthy snacks or with water and fruit, depending on the school, and parents need to be aware of their child's nutritional exposure.

Activity Assessment

> It can no longer be assumed that children will have enough activity in their day to keep them in energy balance.

As in a nutritional review, a review of daily and weekly activities is essential. Decreasing sedentary behavior in children has been associated with improvement in weight status (15).

The number of hours of television time has been associated with obesity (16) and a reduction in television time with reduced obesity (17). Asking the family and child about television, computer, and game and movie time will give an estimate of total "screen" time. The number and type of food advertisements on television has been linked to childhood risk of overweight both in the United States and in Europe (18). In addition, the presence of a television in the child's bedroom is a risk factor for obesity (19).

Outdoor time is also a measure of total activity; many children do not go outdoors during the week except for recess at school. Recess and physical education at school are activity opportunities, but many times children are not moving during the entire session. Issues such as community access to playgrounds, safety, cost, and transportation to sports activities may all be limiting factors for children and families. Family activities also play an important role in either limiting or encouraging a child to become active. Inquiring into these leisure pastimes will help in evaluating opportunities for change.

Also important are any medical or physical limitations a child may have to increasing physical activity. Conditions such as asthma and deconditioning are common reasons children and parents may limit activity. Sleep apnea presenting as daytime tiredness may also interfere with activity during the day. Motor deficits and developmental delay can present special challenges as families work to increase activity. Children who are depressed or anxious often may be reluctant to participate in peer activities and need help and encouragement to change activity patterns.

Family, Psychosocial, and Environmental Assessment

Family-based change is key in helping the child or adolescent attain a healthy weight. Family members are asked to "buy into" lifestyle change. Providing necessary information about obesity with its related comorbidities and recommending treatment and options for lifestyle change are important elements of intervention. Stepwise implementation of change with support for setbacks, is vital in helping families learn how to manage risk factors.

In addition to working together, families must be able to assess the nutritional and activity environment both inside and outside the home. They must learn to pay attention to day care and school menus, snacks, and activity opportunities offered at school and after school. Moreover, eating out at restaurants and in other social settings needs to be addressed. For families and children to accomplish lifestyle change, they will need to develop the decision-making skills necessary to functional optimally in their nutrition and activity environment.

Temperament, parenting style, and family interactions may all influence the family's ability to manage healthy nutrition and activity for the child. Helping families work through behavioral issues, which may arise during treatment, enables the process of change.

Focusing on healthier eating and supporting family-based change are more helpful than calorie counting. There are families, however, who want a more structured nutritional plan, and referral to a dietitian can be helpful.

In any plan to address obesity in a child, ongoing support from extended family and physician is crucial. Although the overall goal is return to a healthy weight and energy balance along with resolution of obesity-related comorbidities, goals are tailored to the child's needs and are incremental to allow for success at implementation. Examples of goals are listed in Table 5.2.

FAMILY-BASED LIFESTYLE CHANGE

There are several keys to helping the family make lifestyle change (1):

1. Provide the information the family needs to make health-based decisions.
2. Meet the family where they are. Each family will be at a unique point in their readiness to change, resources, and skills. It is important to recognize and acknowledge that change can start at any point.

TABLE 5.2. *Examples of goals to address in childhood obesity*

Slowing of weight gain
Weight stability
Weight loss
Implementation of agreed-on nutritional/activity change
Improvement in metabolic status
Improvement in comorbidity
Improvement in physical functioning
Improved self-esteem

3. Reaffirm what the family can and does do in support of their and their child's health. This can lay the groundwork for the family's confidence in attempting the next change.
4. Recommend several changes that could be made and have the patient and/or parents decide on which ones they think they could tackle first.
5. Involve the whole family in goal setting and in implementing the decided on change.
6. Self-monitoring of behavior can be a valuable tool to increase the family's awareness of the changes they are making; families may want to keep track of their success in altering specific behaviors, such as reducing the number of times they eat out, decreasing portion sizes, or improving the quality of snacks.
7. Setbacks are a normal part of working on lifestyle change. Encouraging self-monitoring and helping the child and family deal with inevitable setbacks is an important part of ongoing treatment.
8. At return visits, the child and family's progress is assessed and praised, and goals are reaffirmed or modified.

CASE

Initial Presentation

SB is a 6-year-old girl you have cared for in your practice since she was an infant. It is time for her yearly well check. When you see SB's growth chart, plotted by your nurse, you notice that she has crossed from the 75th percentile in weight, which she had been steadily following, and is now in the 90th. Her height is still at the 75th percentile and is nicely following the curve. Her weight is now 56 lb (90th percentile) and her height is 47 in. (75th percentile), with a BMI at the 91st percentile. Her blood pressure is 98/53 mm Hg.

You begin by asking her mother how the family has been over the past year since you have seen them. The mother initially says fine but looks upset, and you ask if anything is wrong. She nods and says that she and her husband have just separated and "things have been rough for a while." You express sympathy and ask with whom SB and her brother are living, and the mother says that the children live with her and they see their father one evening a week and every other weekend.

You ask Mrs. B if she has any specific health or behavior concerns about SB, and she says she has been worried about SB's self-esteem. You ask how she became concerned about this, and the mother says that SB has been making negative remarks about herself and her "belly being too big." She also suspects that SB may be getting teased at school. You ask Mrs. B if she has noticed any change in SB's eating or activity level, and she says that SB seems to be hungry a lot and has refused to join the soccer team she played for last year.

You go over the growth chart with Mrs. B and mention that the family could be eating healthier and getting more activity. Mrs. B agrees.

Then you obtain a dietary history from SB. She is eating cereal and milk for breakfast, and her mother is packing her lunch, which consists of a sandwich, fruit, and pretzels. It turns out that SB frequently is trading her pretzels for chips, and her friends may also give her extra snacks from their lunch. In the after school program, SB has juice and crackers for a snack. When she arrives home, her mother cooks dinner, but her mother notes that SB is continuously asking for food and sometimes will sneak food if she is not given something to eat. Both children are drinking juice between meals; the mother does not buy soda, but SB says there is soda at her father's home.

When asked to estimate the amount of screen time SB has, the mother says about 3 hours, mostly television. She does not know how much television time SB has at her father's house.

You review the family history, which is positive for diabetes in a maternal grandmother and cardiovascular disease in a paternal grandfather. SB's review of systems is essentially normal. On physical examination, the only finding, in addition to a BMI at the 91st percentile, is slightly enlarged tonsils.

You ask the mother if she feels ready to make changes in the family's eating and activity. She says she would like to start. You review some of the possibilities, which include decreasing or eliminating juice, reducing television time, and working with SB to distract her when she is hungry. The mother thinks she can decrease the juice intake and try to distract SB but does not think she can work on the television watching. You start by having the mother try not to buy juice for the household and work with SB on other activities she can do when she feels hungry. You ask the mother to document any juice drinking and to come up with a list of activities for SB, with the goal of stabilizing SB's weight until her next visit in 1 month.

Follow-Up

One month later, SB and her mother return. SB has not gained any weight. The mother reports that not only is she not drinking juice but also she has stopped trading food with her friends at school. The mother notes that SB has made fewer negative comments about herself and has seemed less hungry. You encourage SB and her mother to continue the good job they are doing and ask if there is anything else they would like to change. The mother notes that she would like both SB and her brother to watch less television, and you help the mother figure out how she could accomplish this. You have the mother call to check in with SB's weight in 1 month and schedule a revisit in 2 months. You let the mother know that you would be happy to see Mr. B if she wants him to come to the next appointment.

REFERENCES

1. Dietz WH, Robinson TN. Clinical practice: overweight children and adolescents. *N Engl J Med.* 2005;352:2100–2109.
2. Freedman DS, Wang J, Maynard LM, Thornton JC, Mei Z, Pierson RN, Dietz WH, Horlick M. The relation of BMI to fat and fat-free mass in children and adolescents. *Int J Obes Relat Disord.* 2005;29:1–8.
3. Committee on Prevention of Obesity in Children and Youth, Institute of Medicine; Koplan JP, Liverman CT, Kraak VI, eds. *Prevention of childhood obesity: health in the balance.* Washington, DC: National Academies Press; 2005.

4. Goodman E, Whitaker RC. A prospective study of the role of depression in the development and persistence of adolescent obesity. *Pediatrics.* 2002;110:497–504.
5. Barlow SE, Dietz WH. Obesity evaluation and treatment; expert committee recommendations. The Maternal and Child Health Bureau, Health Resources and Services Administration and the Department of Health and Human Services. *Pediatrics.* 1998;102(3):e29.
6. Daniels SR, Arnett DK, Eckel RH, Gidding SS, Hayman LL, Kumanyika S, Robinson TN, Scott BJ, St. Jeor S, Williams CL. Overweight in children and adolescents: pathophysiology, consequences, prevention, and treatment. *Circulation.* 2005;111(15):1999–2012.
7. Krebs NF, Jacobson MS; American Academy of Pediatrics Committee on Nutrition: Prevention of pediatric overweight and obesity. *Pediatrics.* 2003;112:424–430.
8. Ludwig DS, Peterson KE, Gortmaker SL. Relation between consumption of sugar sweetened drinks and childhood obesity: a prospective, observational analysis. *Lancet.* 2001;357:505–508.
9. Ebbeling CB, Feldman HA, Osganian SK, Chomitz VR, Ellenbogen SJ, Ludwig DS. Effects of decreasing sugar sweetened beverage consumption on body weight in adolescents: a randomized controlled pilot study. *Pediatrics.* 2006;117:673–680.
10. Nestle M. Increasing portion sizes in American diets: more calories, more obesity. *J Am Diet Assoc.* 2003;103:39–40.
11. Orlet Fisher J, Rolls BJ, Birch LL. Children's bite size and intake of an entrée are greater with large portions than with age-appropriate or self selected portions. *Am J Clin Nutr.* 2003;77:1164–1170.
12. Bowman SA, Gortmaker SL, Ebbeling CB, Pereira MA, Ludwig DS. Effects of fast-food consumption on energy intake and diet quality among children in a national household survey. *Pediatrics.* 2004;113(1 Pt 10):112–118.
13. Epstein LH, Gordy CC, Raynor HA, Beddome M, Kilanowski CK, Paluch R. Increasing fruit and vegetable intake and decreasing fat and sugar intake in families at risk for childhood obesity. *Obes Res.* 2001;9:171–178.
14. Skinner JD, Bounds W, Carruth BR, Ziegler P. Longitudinal calcium intake is negatively related to children's body fat indexes. *J Am Diet Assoc.* 2003;103:1626–1631.
15. Epstein LH, Paluch RA, Gordy CC, Dorn J. Decreasing sedentary behaviors in treating pediatric obesity. *Arch Pediatr Adolesc Med.* 2000;154:220–226.
16. Gortmaker S, Must A, Sobol A, Peterson K, Colditz G, Dietz W. Television viewing as a cause of increasing obesity among children in the United States, 1986-1990. *Arch Pediatr Adolesc Med.* 1996;150(4):356–362.
17. Robinson TN. Reducing children's television viewing to prevent obesity: a randomized controlled trial. *JAMA.* 1999;282(16):1561–1567.
18. Lobstein T, Dibb S. Evidence of a possible link between obesogenic food advertising and child overweight. *Obes Rev.* 2005;6:203–208.
19. Dennison BA, Erb TA, Jenkins PL. Television viewing and television in bedroom associated with overweight risk among low-income preschool children. *Pediatrics.* 2002;109:1028–1035.

6

Respiratory Complications

Obesity has a profound impact on the respiratory system. Excess adiposity alters structure, affects function, and may influence the metabolic status of the lung. Structurally, excess adipose tissue deposition in and around the pharynx has been implicated in increasing the likelihood of upper airway obstruction (UAO) (1). Abdominal fat deposition may compromise respiratory excursion (2), and infiltration of adipocytes into the diaphragmatic muscle may alter respiratory mechanics and function (3). The inflammatory state induced by the production of adipokines may exacerbate asthma (4).

> Compromise of the respiratory system by obesity has implications for obesity progression and treatment.

- Children who have sleep-disordered breathing (SDB) are more likely to suffer from tiredness, poor performance in school, deficits in attention and memory, and poor decision making (5–8).
- These deficits all compromise a child's ability to fully participate in activities, which may encourage further weight gain.
- Children who are tired and inattentive may often be labeled "lazy and unmotivated," causing a vicious cycle of discouragement and low self-esteem.
- Obese children who have worsening asthma often have activity restrictions that compromise calorie burning.

The respiratory complications of obesity can also contribute to long-term morbidity. Severe obstructive sleep apnea syndrome (OSAS) can result in pulmonary hypertension, right ventricular enlargement, and heart failure. Left ventricular hypertrophy can occur and is linked to the severity of OSAS (9). Systemic hypertension has also been reported in children as well as adults (10). Some findings suggest that the severity of OSAS is related to that of neurocognitive impairment (5). Finally, respiratory compromise from asthma can lead to inactivity, physical deconditioning, worsening obesity, and chronically impaired lung function.

UPPER AIRWAY OBSTRUCTION

State of the Problem

The effect of obesity on the incidence of UAO in childhood is superimposed on the traditional causes of UAO, such as enlarged tonsils and adenoids, craniofacial anomalies, and hypotonia. Therefore, the spectrum of symptomatology ranges from traditional childhood symptoms in younger aged patients, when tonsillar enlargement is prevalent, to a more adult presentation in the obese adolescent.

Obstructive sleep apnea is estimated to affect 0.7% to 3.4% of all children (11). In one series of obese children, polysomnographic abnormalities were found in 37% of patients studied (12). In obese children referred for snoring or abnormal breathing during sleep, 59% were diagnosed with OSAS (13). Symptoms of UAO may appear at any point in childhood as obesity worsens. Obese infants have been found to have an increased number of 3- to 10-second episodes of airway obstruction, more gross body movements, and more sleep stage shifts than nonobese infants (14).

UAO is a prominent respiratory manifestation of excess adipose tissue accumulation.

Other components of SDB include the following:

- Snoring
- Upper airway resistance syndrome (UARS)
- Upper airway obstruction
- Obesity hypoventilation syndrome (Pickwickian syndrome)

Appreciation of this continuum of SDB is important because sleep disruption, in addition to later hypoxemia and hypercarbia, is thought to account for significant compromise of prefrontal cortex function, which has direct implications for learning and behavior in childhood (8).

Definitions

The following definitions are listed to help clarify the types of respiratory disturbances that are linked to obesity.

- **Sleep-disordered breathing**—Breathing disorders during sleep that range in severity from primary snoring through persistent snoring, UARS, OSAS, and obesity hypoventilation syndrome.

- **Primary snoring**—Snoring that occurs without obstructive apnea, gas exchange abnormalities, or excessive arousals (15).
- **Upper airway resistance syndrome (UARS)**—Snoring with partial UAO that leads to repetitive episodes of increased respiratory efforts ending in arousals. The sleep pattern is disrupted and daytime symptoms may occur. No evidence of apnea, hypopnea, or gas exchange abnormalities can be found on polysomnography (10).
- **Obstructive sleep apnea syndrome (OSAS)**—A disorder of breathing during sleep that in children is characterized by prolonged partial UAO and/or intermittent complete obstruction (obstructive apnea) that disrupts normal ventilation during sleep and normal sleep patterns (15). The condition is characterized by alternating apneic pauses and arousals, often with oxygen desaturation and/or hypercarbia, producing restless sleep and a feeling of fatigue on awakening (15).
- **Obesity hypoventilation syndrome**—Results from continuous partial airway obstruction that leads to paradoxical respiratory efforts, hypercarbia, and often hypoxemia (16).
- **Obstructive apnea**—Cessation of oronasal airflow with continued respiratory effort (17).
- **Hypopnea**—A reduction but not complete cessation of airflow (17), clinically manifested by shallow breathing.
- **Apnea index**—The number of total apnea episodes during sleep plus the number of total hypopnea episodes during sleep divided by the total sleep time in minutes (17).

Etiology

Although not all obese children have SDB, obesity increases the likelihood of SDB, and the more obese a child is, the more likely he or she will be to exhibit some symptoms of sleep disturbance and compromised daytime functioning (13).

It is easy to imagine that excess adipose tissue accumulation in the head, neck, and upper airway can cause narrowing and respiratory compromise (1). In addition, fatty infiltration of the muscles of the hypopharynx and diaphragm may affect muscle function (3). Obesity in adults has been shown to cause decreased chest wall compliance, reduced strength of inspiratory muscles, and a restrictive ventilatory pattern, which predicts hypercapnia (18), and reduced lung volumes have been thought to reflexly induce a reduction in the size of the upper airway (19). Evidence also suggests that the metabolic effects of obesity may contribute to disturbances of respiration during sleep. For example, leptin, an obesity-associated cytokine, has been found to correlate with OSAS, and it decreases when treatment with continuous positive airway pressure (CPAP) is administered (20). Tumor necrosis factor-α

(TNF-α) and interleukin-6 (IL-6) produce sleepiness and fatigue and are both elevated in sleep apnea and obesity (21). The presence of enlarged adenoids and tonsils will exacerbate hypercarbia and hypoxemia in obese children with SDB because the shape of the palate changes, nasal passages are narrowed, the face is flatter and broader, and the glabella is flattened (13).

Clinical Manifestations

Clinical manifestations of SDB can be divided into sleep-related nighttime symptoms, which involve disturbances of breathing and sleep, and daytime symptoms, which involve tiredness and reduced cognitive functioning (Table 6.1).

Obese children with OSAS have shown deficits in memory and learning on standardized tests when compared with obese children without OSAS (5). Even normal weight children with simple snoring showed deficits in attention and lower memory and intelligence scores than nonsnorers, along with reduced performance and verbal and global intelligence quotient (IQ) scores (22). Symptoms of UAO can be confused with those of attention deficit disorder (ADD), and children with UAO may be thought to have ADD or unfortunately may be labeled "lazy" or "unmotivated." In one study of a cross-section of school children, early childhood snoring was associated with poor academic performance in middle school (23). Serious complications of UAO can occur in childhood, such as the following:

- Systemic hypertension
- Pulmonary hypertension
- Cor pulmonale

TABLE 6.1. *Clinical manifestations of sleep-disordered breathing*

Nighttime symptoms	Daytime symptoms
Snoring	Morning headache
Restless sleeping	Daytime tiredness
Heavy or noisy breathing	Napping
Orthopnea/Sleeping sitting up	Poor school performance
Frequent night awakening	Inattentiveness
Enuresis	Short-term memory deficits
Observed apnea	Irritability
Diaphoresis	Increased blood pressure
Cyanosis	

From references 5–8,10,12,15–17.

Obesity hypoventilation syndrome is at one end of the spectrum of respiratory disturbances caused by excess adiposity. It results from the interactions of small lung volume due to relatively mobile chest wall and restriction of diaphragmatic movement due to abdominal fat, which increase the work of breathing (16). This sets up a breathing pattern that is shallow and rapid and reduces the proportion of each breath available for gas exchange (16). The Pickwickian syndrome is marked by an impaired ventilatory response to hypercarbia, which occurs centrally. The exact mechanism of obesity-related hypoventilation is unknown. In leptin-deficient ob/ob mice, a diminished central response to hypercapnia is reversed by administration of leptin (24). This finding may be pertinent to obese patients who, although having high levels of leptin, are leptin resistant (20).

Clinical manifestations of the obesity hypoventilation syndrome (18) are as follows:

- Daytime somnolence, difficulty with arousal from sleep
- Hypercapnia
- Polycythemia
- Right ventricular hypertrophy
- Cyanosis
- Periodic respiration, apneic pauses
- Right ventricular failure associated with alveolar hyperventilation (18)

Total lung capacity, functional residual capacity, and expiratory reserve volume are decreased, resulting in alveolar hypoventilation, arterial hypoxemia, and hypercarbia (18). Ventilation-perfusion mismatches may also occur, and patients so affected may be more susceptible to respiratory compromise when pulmonary infections occur (16). These patients have a complex course and significant morbidity and should be under the care of a specialist.

Evaluation

> Every obese child should be asked about the quality of his or her sleep, and attention paid to any problems in school performance or behavior, as they may be symptoms of SDB.

The physical examination reveals an obese child who may or may not also show evidence of adenotonsillar hypertrophy, such as mouth breathing, nasal obstruction during wakefulness, adenoidal facies, and hypernasal speech. Complications such as systemic hypertension or increased component of the second heart sound, indicative of pulmonary hypertension, may be detected (15).

The "gold standard" of diagnosis of SDB is nighttime polysomnography (7). Although some symptom checklists have proved useful in predicting SDB in the research setting, there has been no large-scale clinical evaluation of these scales (25).

Parental observation, video taping, and audio taping are suggestive but not necessarily predictive of a positive or negative sleep study (7).

Standards of measurement on polysomnography are the following (6):

1. Respiratory effort as assessed by abdominal and chest wall movement
2. Airflow at nose/mouth or both
3. Arterial oxygen saturation via pulse oximetry (noninvasive)
4. Electrocardiographic (ECG) rate and rhythm
5. Electromyography in the anterior tibial region to monitor arousals
6. Electroencephalographic (EEG), electro-oculographic, and electromyographic measurement for sleep staging (6)

If cardiac disease is suspected, a chest radiograph, echocardiogram, and electrocardiogram should be obtained (9).

Treatment

The definitive treatment for obesity-associated SDB is weight loss (26). When indicated, tonsilloadenoidectomy (T & A) is performed. If T & A is not indicated, or if the sleep study is positive after a T & A, CPAP, bilevel airway pressure (BiPAP), or oxygen therapy is used.

1. **Tonsilloadenoidectomy.** Obesity exacerbates UAO due to enlarged tonsils and adenoids (27). Careful attention to postoperative monitoring is important, especially in children with central nervous system (CNS) dysfunction, hypotonia, severe OSAS, age less than 3 years, and craniofacial anomalies in addition to obesity (28). Postoperative morbidity has been more frequently observed in patients with severe preoperative obstructive symptoms, such as daytime somnolence, retractions, choking, cyanosis, frequent waking, and apnea, and in patients with moderately to strongly positive sleep studies, patients in whom surgery was performed urgently, and patients with cardiomegaly (29). Postoperative weight gain is a known effect of T & A in normal weight children and has been reported in obese and morbidly obese children after T & A for obstructive sleep apnea (27).

2. **CPAP.** This has been shown to be an effective treatment for OSAS in children (30). CPAP is accomplished by an electronic device that delivers constant air pressure via a nasal mask, prongs, or nasal pillows, leading to mechanical stenting of the airway and improved functional residual capacity in the lung. CPAP must be titrated in a sleep laboratory and periodically readjusted (15), and children may require behavioral desensitization for effective use (16). Other measures that have been reported to increase compliance include improved mask fit, use of a low-pressure alarm, and frequent clinic visits (30). Side effects of nasal congestion, dryness, rhinorrhea, eye irritation, conjunctivitis, dermatitis, and skin ulceration due to poor mask fit or pressure have been noted (30).

3. **BiPAP.** This is delivered during expiration and inspiration by mask or nasal prongs (31). BiPAP has proved effective in reducing the apnea/hypopnea index and increasing oxygen saturation in obese patients with OSAS (31).

4. **Oxygen therapy.** If oxygen therapy is to be used in children, it should be evaluated during continuous CO_2 monitoring in the sleep laboratory to assess its effect on hypoventilation (15).

5. **Other surgical options.** For patients not responding to the usual treatment, other surgical options may be considered. These patients should be referred to pediatric surgical subspecialists, and options may include uvulopharyngopalatoplasty, craniofacial surgery, and, in severe cases, tracheostomy (15).

Special Situations

Anesthesia

Postsurgical complications have been reported in children with obstructive sleep apnea after T & A, which have included (28):

- Increased snoring
- Increased work of breathing during sleep
- Consistently low oxygen saturation requiring continued repositioning and supplemental oxygen
- Need for nasal CPAP or BiPAP
- Requirement for prolonged intubation
- Need for reintubation

These complications were associated with younger age, more severe apnea, decreased oxygen saturation, and associated medical problems, including hypotonia, morbid obesity, craniofacial abnormalities and upper airway burn, young age, cor pulmonale, respiratory distress index (RDI) greater than 40, or oxygen saturation nadir lower than 70% (28). In a small series of obese patients (14 patients) ages 4 to 15, two patients required overnight BiPAP, one required prolonged intubation, and three required supplemental oxygen after T&A (32).

Prader-Willi Syndrome

In obese Prader-Willi syndrome (PWS) patients, hypercapnic ventilatory responses were blunted compared with those in nonobese PWS patients or obese control subjects. Isocapnic hypoxic ventilatory responses were absent or severely reduced in both obese and nonobese PWS patients (33). There have been case reports of PWS patients treated with growth hormone who experienced obstructive apnea, respiratory infection, and sudden death (34). Such reports would militate against the use of growth hormone in these patients.

ASTHMA

State of the Problem

The rise in childhood obesity since the 1980s has been paralleled by a rise in asthma rates. Asthma and obesity also often occur together (35), and increases in body mass index (BMI) have been associated with a greater incidence of asthma (36).

Weight reduction in obese individuals has been shown to alleviate asthma symptoms (35).

In a longitudinal population-based cohort study adjusted for risk factors, being overweight or obese at age 11 years was associated with a threefold increased risk for persistence of infrequent wheezing after adolescence and with a twofold increased risk for persistence of asthma (37). A study of 5- to 6-year-old children showed that the prevalence of doctor-diagnosed asthma rose with increased BMI; interestingly, this effect was confined to girls (38). In a meta-analysis of overweight and asthma, high body weight in infancy or childhood was linked with a higher incidence of asthma (39). In a study of urban minority children, those with asthma were more likely to be obese than those without, and 30% of the children with asthma had a BMI greater than the 95th percentile, whereas only 12% of the children without asthma were obese (40).

Etiology

The link between obesity and asthma is not entirely clear, although both are associated with chronic inflammatory states. Asthma is a chronic inflammatory disease of the airways that causes recurrent episodes of wheezing, breathlessness, chest tightness, and cough. This inflammation also produces an increase in existing bronchial hyperresponsiveness (41). Obese children may have gastroesophageal reflux as well, which can precipitate wheezing and asthma. Obesity has also been characterized as an inflammatory state (42), and overweight nonasthmatic children have been shown to have a higher susceptibility to exercise-induced bronchospasm (43). In addition, leptin, a proinflammatory cytokine present in higher levels in obese children (42), has also been found in increased levels in normal weight boys with asthma when compared with nonasthmatic controls (44).

Mechanical factors may also contribute to asthmatic symptoms. Lung volumes and thoracic wall distensibility were found to be decreased in obese girls (45), and obesity is associated with a breathing pattern of higher frequencies and lower tidal volumes (35). As a result of this shallower breathing pattern, there is less bronchial smooth muscle stretch and greater muscle stiffness, resulting in more difficulty stretching, muscle fiber shortening, and increased bronchial hyperresponsiveness (35).

Clinical Manifestations

Overweight may contribute to increased severity of asthma and, in a study of inner city black and Hispanic children, was associated with a lower than predicted peak expiratory flow rate. In addition, these obese asthmatic children were reported to miss more school days and receive more medications than nonobese asthmatic children (46). Obese children with and without asthma report more coughing, wheezing, and dyspnea than nonobese children (47). Increased bronchial responsiveness may lead to avoidance of exercise, which can lead to or exacerbate obesity (48).

Evaluation and Treatment

Obese children are at higher risk for asthma and may present with a diagnosis already in place. However, obese children may have a very low level of activity and may not voluntarily report symptoms, so a careful history for asthma, particularly exercise-induced asthma, should be obtained. Care must be taken to identify altered activity patterns, such as dropping out of sports or activities, "slowing down," and losing interest, which might be the result of increased respiratory symptoms such as shortness of breath, chest tightness, and wheezing. Attention to changes in exercise symptoms needs to be maintained over time. As increased physical activity becomes part of a weight management strategy, previously unrecognized respiratory symptoms may emerge.

Asthma treatment should be optimized in all children and is especially critical in obese children. Those who may have decreased physical activity because of asthma symptoms need to feel confident that exercise is safe and possible, and optimal asthma care can provide this support.

ONGOING SUPPORT

1. Children with sleep apnea need ongoing monitoring and support, not only to encourage weight loss but also to monitor progression of symptoms and use of CPAP or BiPAP.
2. Asthma management should be optimized in all children, with attention focused on preventing exacerbations and maximizing pulmonary function to allow for optimal activity.

IMPACT ON WEIGHT MANAGEMENT

OSAS may contribute to worsening of the metabolic and cardiovascular picture associated with obesity. Nocturnal sleep and respiratory disturbances in obese patients with sleep apnea are independent risk factors for hyperinsulinemia (49). SDB may increase the risk of developing the metabolic syndrome (50). Repeated episodes of apnea and hypopnea are known to cause transient elevations in blood pressure during sleep, and daytime blood pressure increases linearly with an increasing apnea/hypopnea index (51). Moreover, OSAS is associated with stroke and heart disease in adults (52).

In adults, SDB has also been associated with increased sympathetic nervous system activity (53), decreased baroreceptor sensitivity (54), accentuated vascular responsiveness (55), and abnormal salt and water metabolism (56), all of which could contribute to hypertension.

An inverse correlation between memory and learning performance and the apnea/hypopnea index was found in morbidly obese children with OSAS (5). Beebe and Gozal (8) have proposed that the effect of OSAS in children, causing sleep disruption and intermittent hypoxemia and hypercarbia, alters cellular and chemical homeostasis that leads to deficits in prefrontal cortex function. Deficits in behavioral inhibition, set shifting, self-regulation of affect and arousal, working memory, analysis/synthesis, and contextual memory, all of which play an important role in executive functioning, can occur (8). Executive functioning has been referred to as the ability to develop and sustain an organized future-oriented and flexible approach to problem situations (8). These are all skills important for participating in therapies to create behavior and lifestyle change involved in obesity treatment.

Asthma is a consideration in any weight management plan. Poorly controlled asthma may preclude the increased activity necessary to achieve improved energy balance. In addition, asthma and exercise asthma may become apparent in an obese child who initiates exercise as part of a weight management plan. Exercise is also important in asthma treatment, and a prescription for exercise has been endorsed for all asthmatic subjects by the American College of Sports Medicine and the American Thoracic Society (57).

REFERENCES

1. Shelton KE, Woodson H, Gay S, Suratt PM. Pharyngeal fat in obstructive sleep apnea. *Am Rev Respir Dis.* 1993;148(2):462–466.
2. Kessler R, Chaouat A, Schinkewitch P, Faller M, Casel S, Krieger J, Weitzenblum E. The obesity-hypoventilation syndrome revisited: a prospective study of 34 consecutive cases. *Chest.* 2001;120(2): 369–376.
3. Fadell E, Richman AD, Ward WW, Hendon JR. Fatty infiltration of the respiratory muscles in the Pickwickian syndrome. *N Engl J Med.* 1962;266(17):861–863.
4. Guler N, Kirerleri E, Ones U, Tamay Z, Salmayenli N, Darendeliler F. Leptin: does it have any role in childhood asthma? *J Allergy Clin Immunol.* 2004;114(2):254–259.
5. Rhoades SK, Shimoda KC, Waid LR, ONeil PM, Oexman MJ, Collop NA, Willi SM. Neurocognitive deficits in morbidly obese children with obstructive sleep apnea. *J Pediatr.* 1995;127(5):741–744.
6. American Thoracic Society Medical Section of the American Lung Association. Cardiorespiratory sleep studies in children. Establishment of normative data and polysomnographic predictors of morbidity. *Am J Respir Crit Care Med.* 1999;160(4):1381–1387.
7. Sterni LM, Tunkel DE. Obstructive sleep apnea in children: an update. *Pediatr Clin North Am.* 2003;50(2):427–443.
8. Beebe DW, Gozal D. Obstructive sleep apnea and the prefrontal cortex: towards a comprehensive model linking nocturnal upper airway obstruction to daytime cognitive and behavioral deficits. *J Sleep Res.* 2002;11(1):1–16.
9. Amin RS, Kimball TR, Bean JA, Jeffries JL, Willging JP, Cotton RT, Witt SA, Glascock BJ, Daniels SR. Left ventricular hypertrophy and abnormal ventricular geometry in children and adolescents with obstructive sleep apnea. *Am J Respir Crit Care Med.* 2002;165(10):1395–1399.

10. Schechter M. Section on Pediatric Pulmonology, Subcommittee on Obstructive Sleep Apnea Syndrome. Technical report: diagnosis and management of childhood obstructive sleep apnea syndrome. *Pediatrics.* 2002;109(4):e69–e98.

11. Nieminen P, Lopponen T, Tolonen U, Lanning P, Knip M, Lopponen H. Growth and biochemical markers of growth in children with snoring and obstructive sleep apnea. *Pediatrics.* 2002;109(4): e55–e61.

12. Mallory GB, Fiser DH, Jackson R. Sleep associated breathing disorders in morbidly obese children and adolescents. *J Pediatr.* 1989;115(6):892–897.

13. Silvestri JM, Weese-Mayer DE, Bass MT, Kenney AS, Hauptman Sa, Pearsall SM. Polysomnography in obese children with a history of sleep-associated breathing disorders. *Pediatr Pulmonol.* 1993; 16(2):124–126.

14. Kahn A, Mozin MJ, Rebuffat E, Sottiaux W, Burniat W, Shephard S, Muller MF. Sleep pattern alterations and brief airway obstructions in overweight infants. *Sleep.* 1989;12(5):430–438.

15. Section on Pediatric Pulmonology, Subcommittee on Obstructive Sleep Apnea Syndrome, American Academy of Pediatrics. Clinical Practice Guideline: diagnosis and management of childhood obstructive sleep apnea syndrome. *Pediatrics.* 2002;109(4):704–712.

16. Riley DJ, Santiago TV, Edelman NH. Complications of obesity—hypoventilation syndrome in childhood. *Am J Dis Child.* 1976;130(6):671–675.

17. Guillenminault C, Korobkin R, Winkle R. A review of 50 children with obstructive sleep apnea syndrome. *Lung.* 1981;159(5):275–287.

18. Burwell CS, Robin ED, Whaley RD, Bickelmann AG. Extreme obesity associated with alveolar hypoventilation—a Pickwickian syndrome. *Am J Med.* 1956;21(5):811–818.

19. Hoffstein V, Zamel N, Phillipson EA. Lung volume dependence of pharyngeal cross-sectional area in patients with obstructive sleep apnea. *Am Rev Respir Dis.* 1984;130(2):175–178.

20. Ip MS, Lam KS, Ho C, Tsang KW, Lam W. Serum leptin and vascular risk factors in obstructive sleep apnea. *Chest.* 2000;118(3):580–586.

21. Vgontzas AN, Papanicolaou DA, Bixler EO, Kales A, Tyson K, Chorousos GP. Elevation of plasma cytokines in disorders of excessive daytime sleepiness and role of sleep disturbance and obesity. *J Clin Endocrinol Metab* 1997;82(5):1313–1316.

22. Blunden S, Lushington K, Kennedy D, Martin J, Dawson D. Behavior and neurocognitive performance in children aged 5-10 years who snore compared to controls. *J Clin Exp Neuropsychol.* 2000;22(5):554–568.

23. Gozal D, Pope DW. Snoring during early childhood and academic performance at ages 13-14. *Pediatrics.* 2001;107(6):1394–1399.

24. Groeben H, Meier S, Brown RH, O'Donnell CP, Mitzner W, Tankersley CG. The effect of leptin on the ventilatory response to hyperoxia. *Exp Lung Res.* 2004;30(7):559–570.

25. Chervin RD, Hedger K, Dillon JE, Pituch KJ. Pediatric Sleep Questionnaire (PSQ) validity and reliability of scales for sleep disordered breathing, snoring, sleepiness and behavior problems. *Sleep Med.* 2000;1(1):21–32.

26. Willi SM, Oexmann MJ, Wright NM, Collop Na, Key LL. The effects of a high protein low-fat ketogenic diet on adolescents with morbid obesity; body composition, blood chemistries; sleep abnormalities. *Pediatrics.* 1998;101(1 Pt 1):61–67.

27. Soultan Z, Wadowski S, Rao M, Kravath RE. Effect of treating obstructive sleep apnea by tonsillectomy and or adenoidectomy on obesity in children. *Arch Pediatr Adolesc Med.* 1999;153(1):33–37.

28. Rosen GM, Muckle RP, Mahowald MW, Goding GS, Ullevig C. Postoperative respiratory compromise in children with obstructive sleep apnea: can it be anticipated? *Pediatrics.* 1994;93(5):784–788.

29. Price SD, Hawkins DB, Kahlstrom EJ. Tonsil and adenoid surgery for airway obstruction: preoperative respiratory morbidity. *Ear Nose Throat J.* 1993;72(8):526–531.

30. Marcus CL, Ward SL, Mallory GB, Rosen CL, Beckerman RC, Weese-Mayer DE, Brouillette RT, Trang HT, Brooks LJ. Use of nasal continuous positive airway pressure as a treatment of childhood obstructive sleep apnea. *J Pediatr.* 1995;127(1):88–94.

31. Padman R, Hyde C, Foster P, Borkowski W. The pediatric use of bilevel positive airway pressure therapy for obstructive sleep apnea syndrome: a retrospective review with analysis of respiratory parameters. *Clin Pediatr.* 2002;41:163–169.

32. Spector A, Scheid S, Hassink S, Deutsch ES, Reilly JS, Cook SP. Adenotonsillectomy in the morbidly obese child. *Int J Pediatr Otorhinolaryngol.* 2003;67(4):359–364.

33. Arens R, Gozal D, Omlin KJ, Livingston FR, Liu J, Keens TG, Ward SL. Hypoxic and hypercapnic ventilatory responses in Prader-Willi syndrome. *J Appl Physiol.* 1994;77(5):2224–2230.

34. Van Vliet G, Deal CL, Crock PA, Robitaille Y, Oligny LL. Sudden death in growth hormone-treated children with Prader-Willi syndrome. *J Pediatr.* 2004;144(1):129–131.
35. Weiss S, Shore S. Obesity and Asthma Direction for Research NHLBI Workshop. *Am J Respir Crit Care Med.* 2004;169;963–968.
36. Chinn S, Rona RJ. Can the increase in body mass index explain the rising trend in asthma in children? *Thorax.* 2001;56(11):845–850.
37. Guerra S, Wright AL, Morgan WJ, Sherill DL, Holberg CJ, Martinez FD. Persistence of asthma symptoms during adolescence role of obesity and age at the onset of puberty. *Am J Respir Crit Care Med.* 2004;170(1):78–85.
38. von Kries R, Hermann M, Grunert VP, von Mutius E. Is obesity a risk factor for childhood asthma. *Allergy.* 2001;56(4):318–322.
39. Flaherman V, Rutherford GW. A meta analysis of high weight on asthma. *Arch Dis Child.* 2006;91(4):334–339.
40. Gennuso J, Epstein LH, Paluch RA, Cerny F. The relationship between asthma and obesity in urban minority children and adolescents. *Arch Pediatr Adolesc Med.* 1998;152(12):1197–1200.
41. Szilagyi PG, Kemper KJ. Management of chronic childhood asthma in the primary care office. *Pediatr Ann.* 1999;28(1):43–52.
42. Loffreda S, Yang SQ, Lin HZ, Karp CL Brengman ML, Wang DJ, Klein AS, Bulkley GB, Bao C, Noble PW, Lane MD, Diehl AM. Leptin regulates proinflammatory immune responses *FASEB J.* 1998;12(1):57–65.
43. Kaplan TA, Montana E. Exercise induced bronchospasm in nonasthmatic obese children. *Clin Pediatr (Phil).* 1993;32(4):220–225.
44. Guler N, Kirerleri E, Ones U, Tamay Z, Salmayenli N, Darendeliler F. Leptin: does it have any role in childhood asthma? *J Allergy Clin Immunol.* 2004;114(2):254–259.
45. Fung KP, Lau SP, Chow OK, Lee J, Wong TW. Effects of overweight on lung function. *Arch Dis Child.* 1990;65(5):512–515.
46. Luder E, Melnik TA, DiMaio M. Association of being overweight with greater asthma symptoms in inner city black and Hispanic children. *J Pediatr.* 1998;132(4):699–703.
47. del Rio-Navaro B, Cisneros-Rivero M, Berber Eslava A, Epinola-Reyna G, Sienre-Monge J J L. Exercise induced bronchospasm in asthmatic and non-asthmatic obese children. *Allergol Immunopathol (Madr).* 2000;28(1):5–11.
48. Romieu I, Mannino DM, Redd SC, McGeehin MA. Dietary intake, physical activity, body mass index and childhood asthma in the Third National Health and Nutrition Survey (NHANES III). *Pediatr Pulmonol.* 2004;38(1):31–42.
49. Vgontzas AN, Papanicolaou DA, Bixler EO, Hopper K, Lotsikas A, Lin HM, Kales A, Chrousos G. Sleep apnea and daytime sleepiness and fatigue relation to visceral obesity, insulin resistance and hypercytokinemia. *J Clin Endocrinol Metab.* 2000;85(3):1151–1158.
50. Couglin S, Calverley P, Wilding J. Sleep disordered breathing—a new component of syndrome X. *Obes Rev.* 2001;2(4):267–274.
51. Young T, Peppard P, Palta M, Hla KM, Finn L, Morgan B, Skatrud J. Population based study of sleep disordered breathing as a risk factor for hypertension. *Arch Intern Med.* 1997;157(15):1746–1752.
52. Partinen M. Ischaemic stroke snoring and obstructive sleep apnea. *J Sleep Res.* 1995;4(S1):156–159.
53. Carlson JT, Hedner J, Elam M, Ejnell H, Sellgren J, Wallin BG. Augmented resting sympathetic activity in awake patients with obstructive sleep apnea. *Chest.* 1993;103(6):1763–1768.
54. Carlson JT, Hedner JA, Sellgren J, Elam M, Wallin BG. Depressed baroreceptor sensitivity in patients with obstructive sleep apnea. *Am J Respir Crit Care Med.* 1996;154(5):1490–1496.
55. Hedner JA, Wilcox I, Laks L, Grunstein RR, Sullivan CE. A specific and potent effect of hypoxia in patients with sleep apnea. *Am Rev Respir Dis.* 1992;146(5 Pt 1):1240–1245.
56. Rodenstein DO, D'Odemont JP, Pieters T, Auber-Tulkens G. Diurnal and nocturnal diuresis and natriuresis in obstructive sleep apnea. *Am Rev Respir Dis.* 1992;145(6):1367–1371.
57. Lucas SR, Platts-Mills TA. Physical activity and exercise in asthma; Relevance to etiology and treatment. *J Allergy Clin Immunol.* 2005;115(5):928–934.

7

Cardiovascular Complications

OVERVIEW

Heart disease has become a major cause of morbidity and mortality worldwide. Cardiovascular disease accounted for 29.2% of deaths (16.7 million individuals) across the globe in 2003. Once thought to be a disease of developed countries, it is expected to become the leading cause of death in developing countries by 2010. Approximately 80% of cardiovascular disease deaths occur in low- and middle-income countries: "This rise in cardiovascular disease reflects a shift in dietary habits, physical activity levels and tobacco consumption as a result of industrialization, urbanization, economic development and food market globalization" (1). The major biologic risk factors for cardiovascular disease are hypertension, elevated cholesterol, type 2 diabetes, and obesity. The epidemiologic and biologic risk for cardiovascular disease begins in childhood, and the full effect of risk exposure in the population has yet to occur (1). The increasing obesity epidemic points to the alarming future of cardiovascular disease in the young adult and adult population.

Cardiovascular disease risk is increased when children become obese.

Obesity was among the risk factors, which included increased low-density lipoprotein (LDL) and cholesterol, hypertension, and smoking, that were linked to arterial plaque formation in boys as young as 15 years (2). Specific risk factors for cardiovascular disease, high blood pressure, dyslipidemia, *and* elevated body mass index (BMI) in childhood, are associated with coronary artery lesions (3). Obesity-related comorbidities of obstructive sleep apnea, left ventricular hypertrophy, and insulin resistance also contribute to risk of cardiovascular morbidity in obese children and adolescents (4).

State of the Problem

Risk factors for cardiovascular disease cluster in obese individuals. In an analysis of coronary heart disease risk factors among obese children, excess adiposity was associated with the following:

- Increased triglycerides
- Increased LDL cholesterol
- Decreased high-density lipoprotein (HDL) cholesterol
- Increased insulin (5)
- Increased C-reactive protein (CRP) (6,7)
- Increased plasminogen activator inhibitor type I (8)
- Increased homocysteine levels (7,9)
- Decreased adiponectin (7)

In the Bogalusa Heart Study (10), clusters of cardiovascular risk factors (LDL cholesterol >130 mg/dL, triglyceride >130 mg/dL, HDL cholesterol <35 mg/dL, elevated insulin level, systolic or diastolic blood pressure >95th percentile) were more common in children with BMI greater than the 95th percentile. Specific risk clusters may exist within the population of overweight and obese children and adolescents.

Visceral adiposity is reflected in increased waist circumference. Obese children with increased waist circumference have higher mean triglyceride level, mean LDL cholesterol level, glucose level, insulin level, and blood pressure than obese children with lower waist circumference (11).

Adding to the overall risk of cardiovascular disease in obese children is a significant level of physical deconditioning, which has been found in children and adolescents with BMI greater than 40 (12). In an analysis of data from the National Health and Nutrition Examination Survey III (NHANES III), CRP was elevated in children with a BMI greater than the 95th percentile (20.6% of boys and 18.7% of girls) (13) and has been inversely related to levels of physical fitness in boys (14).

Etiology

Vascular endothelial dysfunction, a precursor of atherosclerosis, may be the earliest manifestation of cardiovascular risk in children (15). Children with a history of low birth weight had diminished vascular reactivity compared with normal weight peers, indicating that this may be another effect of the intrauterine environment (16). Childhood obesity is also associated with peripheral vascular dysfunction, the severity of the dysfunction increasing with BMI. Obese children also have a greater carotid intimal medial thickness compared with normal weight children (17). Cardiovascular risk factors can increase along the entire trajectory of childhood.

Population studies have shown that a connection exists between low birth weight and cardiovascular disease (18), diabetes (19), stroke (20), and hypertension (21). Low birth weight has also been linked to risk factors for cardiovascular disease, including obesity, insulin resistance, and impaired glucose tolerance, and is independent of gestational length, smoking, alcohol consumption, and socioeconomic status (22).

Individuals born small for gestational age have been found to have a number of metabolic differences from their normal weight counterparts, which may begin to explain their increased risk for cardiovascular morbidity. Undernutrition in the intrauterine environment may "program" the fetus to respond differently to extrauterine life, particularly if there is an overabundance of available calories, and rapid catch-up growth occurs (23). The highest rate of development of type 2 diabetes occurred in individuals who had low birth weight and increased postnatal growth (24). Early morning fasting cortisol levels in adults increased with lower birth weights, independent of age, BMI, or changes in cortisol binding globulin (25). Fasting cortisol also correlated with current blood pressure, fasting and 2-hour plasma glucose concentration after a glucose tolerance test, plasma triglyceride levels, and insulin resistance (26).

HYPERTENSION

State of the Problem

Worldwide, high blood pressure is estimated to cause 7.1 million deaths, about 13% of total mortality. Blood pressure usually increases steadily with age. Factors associated with hypertension include excess salt intake, lack of exercise, and obesity (27). Children and adolescents with hypertension have an increased risk of hypertension as adults (28,29). In a population study of school-aged children, in whom hypertension was defined as blood pressure greater than the 95th percentile for age and gender, the strongest determinant of essential hypertension in all ethnic groups was BMI percentile (30).

In a study of primary care pediatric patients between the ages of 2 and 19 years, there was a significant correlation between increasing BMI and both systolic and diastolic blood pressure in all age groups (31).

Definitions

- **Childhood/adolescent hypertension**—Systolic and/or diastolic blood pressure greater than the 95th percentile on repeated measurement.
- **Prehypertension**—Systolic and/or diastolic hypertension between the 90th and 95th percentiles. Ambulatory blood pressure monitoring may be useful in situations of "white coat hypertension" (32).

Measuring Blood Pressure

The inflatable bladder of a blood pressure cuff should cover 80% to 100% of the circumference of the arm, with a width-to-length ratio of 1:2. Blood pressure will be overestimated with a cuff that is too small and underestimated with one too large (32) (Table 7.1). Oscillometric blood pressure equipment measures mean arterial pressure, then calculates systolic and diastolic pressures. The algorithms used in these calculations differ for different devices, and measurement can vary widely (33).

The relationship between blood pressure and cardiovascular disease is continuous. Postmortem studies of children and adolescents have demonstrated significant correlations between the level of blood pressure and the presence of atherosclerotic lesions in the aorta and coronary arteries (32).

TABLE 7.1. *Recommended dimensions for blood pressure cuff bladders*

Age range	Width (cm)	Length (cm)	Maximum arm circumference, (cm)[a]
Newborn	4	8	10
Infant	6	12	15
Child	9	18	22
Small adult	10	24	26
Adult	13	30	34
Large adult	16	38	44
Thigh	20	42	52

[a]Calculated so that the bladder would still be able to encircle the largest arm by at least 80%.
Reprinted with permission from National High Blood Pressure Education Program Working Group on High Blood Pressure in Children and Adolescents. The fourth report on the diagnosis, evaluation, and treatment of high blood pressure in children and adolescents. *Pediatrics.* 2004;114:555–576.

In adults, mortality from cardiovascular disease doubles for every 20 mm Hg systolic or 10 mm Hg diastolic blood pressure increase above normal (34). In a study of school-aged children, those with a BMI less than 85% had a prevalence of hypertension of only 2.6% compared with 10.7% in those with a BMI greater than the 95th percentile. The rise in blood pressure with BMI was continuous (30). Systolic blood pressure showed a progressive increase with BMI percentile, whereas no such association was found between diastolic blood pressure and BMI (30). In a longitudinal population study, the effect of childhood BMI on cardiovascular risk factors in adulthood was mediated through the association of childhood BMI with later adult BMI (35). Significant correlations among plasma insulin and systolic blood pressure, diastolic blood pressure, and triglyceride levels have been found in obese children and adolescents (36). In addition, childhood levels of blood pressure have been linked with carotid intimal medial thickness (37) and large artery compliance (38) in young adults.

Etiology

Several basic mechanisms have been proposed to explain obesity-related hypertension. Insulin has an antinatriuretic effect on the kidney via a direct influence on the renal tubule (39). Increased sympathetic stimulation and/or increased activity of the renin-angiotensin system may also contribute to greater sodium resorption as well as increased vasoconstriction (40). Compression of tubules and vasa recta in the renal medulla may also result in greater sodium resorption in obesity (41). Moreover, obese children have increased aldosterone levels (41). Similar to findings in adults, forearm blood flow and forearm vascular resistance have been noted to increase in obese compared with normal weight children (42). A recent study showed that mean blood pressure rose in obese children during exercise and mental stress while forearm blood flow decreased (42). These changes were reversed by an intervention of diet plus exercise training (42).

Leptin may also be involved in the development of obesity-induced hypertension by mediating increased sympathoactivation. In addition, leptin adversely shifts the renal pressure-natriuresis curve, leading to relative sodium retention (43).

Evaluation

The "Fourth Report on the Diagnosis, Evaluation and Treatment of High Blood Pressure in Children and Adolescents" has recommended obtaining a fasting lipid panel for all overweight children with a blood pressure at the 90th percentile or greater, given that both elevated blood pressure and dyslipidemia dramatically increase the risk for cardiovascular disease (36).

Auscultation is the recommended method of blood pressure measurement in children. Elevated blood pressure must be confirmed on repeat visits before diagnosing hypertension in a child (36) (Tables 7.2, 7.3, and 7.4).

Obesity does not rule out other reasons for hypertension, and evaluation for other possible causes should be undertaken as indicated.

Treatment

Control of hypertension in adults reduces morbidity and mortality (32). Weight loss has been shown to reduce blood pressure in adults (44), and weight loss of at least 1 BMI unit over a year has been shown to reduce morbidity (45). Weight loss in children was associated with an improvement in systolic and diastolic blood pressure, LDL cholesterol, triglycerides, and insulin resistance with increased HDL cholesterol, if the body mass index standard deviation score (SDS-BMI) decreased by at least 0.5 over 1 year (46).

The National High Blood Pressure Education Program Working Group on High Blood Pressure has recommended that childhood/adolescent hypertension be treated with weight loss secondary to lifestyle intervention and by pharmacologic therapy as needed (36). Increased physical activity and increased fruit, vegetable, and dairy intake are also recommended. If pharmacologic therapy is indicated, treatment should be initiated with a single drug. Recommended acceptable drug classes for children include angiotensin-converting enzyme (ACE) inhibitors, angiotensin receptor blockers, beta-blockers, calcium channel blockers, and diuretics (36).

The panel recommends that "the goal for antihypertensive treatment in children should be reduction of BP to <95th percentile unless concurrent conditions are present, in which case BP should be lowered to <90th percentile. A definite indication for initiating pharmacologic therapy should be ascertained before a drug is prescribed" (36).

Table 7.4 lists the indications for use of antihypertensive drugs in children as recommended by the National High Blood Pressure Education Program Working Group on High Blood Pressure in Children and Adolescents. Additional details regarding pharmacologic therapy are outlined in the group's report (36).

Ongoing monitoring of target organ damage and drug side effects should be part of the care plan for children with hypertension. Periodic monitoring of electrolytes

Text continued on page 74.

TABLE 7.2. Blood pressure levels for boys by age and height percentile

Age (y)	Blood pressure percentile[a]	Systolic blood pressure (mm Hg) Percentile of height							Diastolic blood pressure (mm Hg) Percentile of height						
		5th	10th	25th	50th	75th	90th	95th	5th	10th	25th	50th	75th	90th	95th
1	50th	80	81	83	85	87	88	89	34	35	36	37	38	39	39
	90th	94	95	97	99	100	102	103	49	50	51	52	53	53	54
	95th	98	99	101	103	104	106	106	54	54	55	56	57	58	58
	99th	105	106	108	110	112	113	114	61	62	63	64	65	66	66
2	50th	84	85	87	88	90	92	92	39	40	41	42	43	44	44
	90th	97	99	100	102	104	105	106	54	55	56	57	58	58	59
	95th	101	102	104	106	108	109	110	59	59	60	61	62	63	63
	99th	109	110	111	113	115	117	117	66	67	68	69	70	71	71
3	50th	86	87	89	91	93	94	95	44	44	45	46	47	48	48
	90th	100	101	103	105	107	108	109	59	59	60	61	62	63	63
	95th	104	105	107	109	110	112	113	63	63	64	65	66	67	67
	99th	111	112	114	116	118	119	120	71	71	72	73	74	75	75
4	50th	88	89	91	93	95	96	97	47	48	49	50	51	51	52
	90th	102	103	105	107	109	110	111	62	63	64	65	66	66	67
	95th	106	107	109	111	112	114	115	66	67	68	69	70	71	71
	99th	113	114	116	118	120	121	122	74	75	76	77	78	78	79
5	50th	90	91	93	95	96	98	98	50	51	52	53	54	55	55
	90th	104	105	106	108	1110	111	112	65	66	67	68	69	69	70
	95th	108	109	110	112	114	115	116	69	70	71	72	73	74	74
	99th	115	116	118	120	121	123	123	77	78	79	80	81	81	82
6	50th	91	92	94	96	98	99	100	53	53	54	55	56	57	57
	90th	105	106	108	110	111	113	113	68	68	69	70	71	72	72
	95th	109	110	112	114	115	117	117	72	72	73	74	75	76	76
	99th	116	117	119	121	123	124	125	80	80	81	82	83	84	84

Age	BP Percentile	SBP							DBP						
7	50th	92	94	95	97	99	100	101	55	55	56	57	58	59	59
	90th	106	107	109	111	113	114	115	70	70	71	72	73	74	74
	95th	110	111	113	115	117	118	119	74	74	75	76	77	78	78
	99th	117	118	120	122	124	125	126	82	82	83	84	85	86	86
8	50th	94	95	97	99	100	102	102	56	57	58	59	60	60	61
	90th	107	109	110	112	114	115	116	71	72	72	73	74	75	76
	95th	111	112	114	116	118	119	120	75	76	77	78	79	79	80
	99th	119	120	122	123	125	127	127	83	84	85	86	87	87	88
9	50th	95	96	98	100	102	103	104	57	58	59	60	61	61	62
	90th	109	110	112	114	115	117	118	72	73	74	75	76	76	77
	95th	113	114	116	118	119	121	121	76	77	78	79	80	81	81
	99th	120	121	123	125	127	128	129	84	85	86	87	88	88	89
10	50th	97	98	100	102	103	105	106	58	59	60	61	61	62	63
	90th	111	112	114	115	117	119	119	73	73	74	75	76	77	78
	95th	115	116	117	119	121	122	123	77	78	79	80	81	81	82
	99th	122	123	125	127	128	130	130	85	86	86	88	88	89	90
11	50th	99	100	102	104	105	107	107	59	59	60	61	62	63	63
	90th	113	114	115	117	119	120	121	74	74	75	76	77	78	78
	95th	117	118	119	121	123	124	125	78	78	79	80	81	82	82
	00th	124	125	127	129	130	132	132	86	86	87	88	89	90	90
12	50th	101	102	104	106	108	109	110	59	60	61	62	63	63	64
	90th	115	116	118	120	121	123	123	74	75	75	76	77	78	79
	95th	119	120	122	123	125	127	127	78	79	80	81	82	82	83
	99th	126	127	129	131	133	134	135	86	87	88	89	90	90	91
13	50th	104	105	106	108	110	111	112	60	60	61	62	63	64	64
	90th	117	118	120	122	124	125	126	75	75	76	77	78	79	79
	95th	121	122	124	126	128	129	130	79	79	80	81	82	83	83
	99th	128	130	131	133	135	136	137	87	87	88	89	90	91	91

(continued)

TABLE 7.2. Blood pressure levels for boys by age and height percentile (continued)

Age (y)	Blood pressure percentile[a]	Systolic blood pressure (mm Hg) Percentile of Height							Diastolic blood pressure (mm Hg) Percentile of Height						
		5th	10th	25th	50th	75th	90th	95th	5th	10th	25th	50th	75th	90th	95th
14	50th	106	107	109	111	113	114	115	60	61	62	63	64	65	65
	90th	120	121	123	125	126	128	128	75	76	77	78	79	79	80
	95th	124	125	127	128	130	132	132	80	80	81	82	83	84	84
	99th	131	132	134	136	138	139	140	87	88	89	90	91	92	92
15	50th	109	110	112	113	115	117	117	61	62	63	64	65	66	66
	90th	122	124	125	127	129	130	131	76	77	78	79	80	80	81
	95th	126	127	129	131	133	134	135	81	81	82	83	84	85	85
	99th	134	135	136	138	140	142	142	88	89	90	91	92	93	93
16	50th	111	112	114	116	118	119	120	63	63	64	65	66	67	67
	90th	125	126	128	130	131	133	134	78	78	79	80	81	82	82
	95th	129	130	132	134	135	137	137	82	83	83	84	85	86	87
	99th	136	137	139	141	143	144	145	90	90	91	92	93	94	94
17	50th	114	115	116	118	120	121	122	65	66	66	67	68	69	70
	90th	127	128	130	132	134	135	136	80	80	81	82	83	84	84
	95th	131	132	134	136	138	139	140	84	85	86	87	87	88	89
	99th	139	140	141	143	145	146	147	92	93	93	94	95	96	97

The 90th percentile is 1.28 SD, the 95th percentile is 1.645 SD, and the 99th percentile is 2.326 SD over the mean.

Reprinted with permission from National High Blood Pressure Education Program Working Group on High Blood Pressure in Children and Adolescents. The fourth report on the diagnosis, evaluation, and treatment of high blood pressure in children and adolescents. *Pediatrics.* 2004;114: 555–576.

TABLE 7.3. Blood pressure for girls by age and height percentile

Age (y)	Blood pressure percentile[a]	Systolic blood pressure (mm Hg) Percentile of height							Diastolic blood pressure (mm Hg) Percentile of height						
		5th	10th	25th	50th	75th	90th	95th	5th	10th	25th	50th	75th	90th	95th
1	50th	83	84	85	86	88	89	90	38	39	39	40	41	41	42
	90th	97	97	98	100	101	102	103	52	53	53	54	55	55	56
	95th	100	101	102	104	105	106	107	56	57	57	58	59	59	60
	99th	108	108	109	111	112	113	114	64	64	65	65	66	67	67
2	50th	85	85	87	88	89	91	91	43	44	44	44	45	46	47
	90th	98	99	100	101	103	104	105	57	58	58	59	60	61	61
	95th	102	103	104	105	107	108	109	61	62	62	63	64	65	65
	99th	109	110	111	112	114	115	116	69	69	70	70	71	72	72
3	50th	86	87	88	89	91	92	93	47	48	48	49	50	50	51
	90th	100	100	102	103	104	106	106	61	62	62	63	64	64	65
	95th	104	104	105	107	108	109	110	65	66	66	67	68	68	69
	99th	111	111	113	114	115	116	117	73	73	74	74	75	76	76
4	50th	88	88	90	91	92	94	94	50	50	51	52	52	53	54
	90th	101	102	103	104	106	107	108	64	64	65	66	67	67	68
	95th	105	106	107	108	110	111	112	68	68	69	70	71	71	72
	99th	112	113	114	115	117	118	119	76	76	76	77	78	79	79
5	50th	89	90	91	93	94	95	96	52	53	53	54	55	55	56
	90th	103	103	105	106	107	109	109	66	67	67	68	69	69	70
	95th	107	107	108	110	111	112	113	70	71	71	72	73	73	74
	99th	114	114	116	117	118	120	120	78	78	79	79	80	81	81
6	50th	91	92	93	94	96	97	98	54	54	55	56	56	57	58
	90th	104	105	106	108	109	110	111	68	68	69	70	70	71	72
	95th	108	109	110	111	113	114	115	72	72	73	74	74	75	76
	99th	115	116	117	119	120	121	122	80	80	80	81	82	83	83

(continued)

TABLE 7.3. Blood pressure for girls by age and height percentile (continued)

Age (y)	Blood pressure percentile[a]	Systolic blood pressure (mm Hg) Percentile of height							Diastolic blood pressure (mm Hg) Percentile of height						
		5th	10th	25th	50th	75th	90th	95th	5th	10th	25th	50th	75th	90th	95th
7	50th	93	93	95	96	97	99	99	55	56	56	57	58	58	59
	90th	106	107	108	109	111	112	113	69	70	70	71	72	72	73
	95th	110	111	112	113	115	116	116	73	74	74	75	76	76	77
	99th	117	118	119	120	122	123	124	81	81	82	82	83	84	84
8	50th	95	95	96	98	99	100	101	57	57	57	58	59	60	60
	90th	108	109	110	111	113	114	114	71	71	71	72	73	74	74
	95th	112	112	114	115	116	118	118	75	75	75	76	77	78	78
	99th	119	120	121	122	123	125	125	82	82	83	83	84	85	86
9	50th	96	97	98	100	101	102	103	58	58	58	59	60	61	61
	90th	110	110	112	113	114	116	116	72	72	72	73	74	75	75
	95th	114	114	115	117	118	119	120	76	76	76	77	78	79	79
	99th	121	121	123	124	125	127	127	83	83	84	84	85	86	87
10	50th	98	99	100	102	103	104	105	59	59	59	60	61	62	62
	90th	112	112	114	115	116	118	118	73	73	73	74	75	76	76
	95th	116	116	117	119	120	121	122	77	77	77	78	79	80	80
	99th	123	123	125	126	127	129	129	84	84	85	86	86	87	88
11	50th	100	101	102	103	105	106	107	60	60	60	61	62	63	63
	90th	114	114	116	117	118	119	120	74	74	74	75	76	77	77
	95th	118	118	119	121	122	123	124	78	78	78	79	80	81	81
	99th	125	125	126	128	129	130	131	85	85	86	87	87	88	89
12	50th	102	103	104	105	107	108	109	61	61	61	62	63	64	64
	90th	116	116	117	119	120	121	122	75	75	75	76	77	78	78
	95th	119	120	121	123	124	125	126	79	79	79	80	81	82	82
	99th	127	127	128	130	131	132	133	86	86	87	88	88	89	90

Age (Year)	BP Percentile	SBP 5%	SBP 10%	SBP 25%	SBP 50%	SBP 75%	SBP 90%	SBP 95%	DBP 5%	DBP 10%	DBP 25%	DBP 50%	DBP 75%	DBP 90%	DBP 95%
13	50th	104	105	106	107	109	110	110	62	62	62	63	63	64	65
	90th	117	118	119	121	122	123	124	76	76	76	77	77	78	79
	95th	121	122	123	124	126	127	128	80	80	80	81	81	82	83
	99th	128	129	130	132	133	134	135	87	87	88	89	89	90	91
14	50th	106	106	107	109	110	111	112	63	63	63	64	64	65	66
	90th	119	120	121	122	124	125	125	77	77	77	78	78	79	80
	95th	123	123	125	126	127	129	129	81	81	81	82	82	83	84
	99th	130	131	132	133	135	136	136	88	88	89	90	90	91	92
15	50th	107	108	109	110	111	113	113	64	64	64	65	66	67	67
	90th	120	121	122	123	125	126	127	78	78	78	79	79	80	81
	95th	124	125	125	127	129	130	131	82	82	82	83	83	84	85
	99th	131	132	133	134	136	137	138	89	89	90	91	91	92	93
16	50th	108	108	110	111	112	114	114	64	64	65	66	66	67	68
	90th	121	122	123	124	126	127	128	78	78	79	80	80	81	82
	95th	125	126	127	128	130	131	132	82	82	83	84	85	85	86
	99th	132	133	134	135	137	138	139	90	90	90	91	92	93	93
17	50th	108	109	110	111	113	114	115	64	65	65	66	67	67	68
	90th	122	122	123	125	126	127	128	78	79	79	80	81	81	82
	95th	125	126	127	129	130	131	132	82	83	83	84	85	85	86
	99th	133	133	134	136	137	138	139	90	90	91	91	92	93	93

[a] The 90th percentile is 1.28 SD, the 95th percentile is 1.645 SD, and the 99th percentile is 2.326 SD over the mean.

Reprinted with permission from National High Blood Pressure Education Program Working Group on High Blood Pressure in Children and Adolescents. The fourth report on the diagnosis, evaluation, and treatment of high blood pressure in children and adolescents. *Pediatrics.* 2004;114: 555–576.

TABLE 7.4. *Indications for antihypertensive drug therapy in children*

Symptomatic hypertension	Diabetes (types 1 and 2)
Secondary hypertension	Persistent hypertension despite
Hypertensive target-organ damage	nonpharmacologic measures

Reprinted with permission from National High Blood Pressure Education Program Working Group on High Blood Pressure in Children and Adolescents. The fourth report on the diagnosis, evaluation, and treatment of high blood pressure in children and adolescents. *Pediatrics.* 2004; 114:555–576.

in children treated with ACE inhibitor or diuretics should be performed. Specific attention to contraindications (e.g., ACE inhibitors are contraindicated for use during pregnancy) and continued counseling regarding lifestyle change are critical (36). Screening for additional comorbidities of obesity should be included in the treatment and care plan. Counseling regarding other cardiovascular risk factors, such as smoking and alcohol use, is important and should begin early. If blood pressure responds to changes in lifestyle, that is, weight loss and increased physical activity, pharmacologic therapy could be tapered (36).

A complete discussion and recommendations for treatment of hypertension in children and adolescents are found in "The Fourth Report on the Diagnosis, Evaluation, and Treatment of High Blood Pressure in Children and Adolescents" (36) (Table 7.5).

DYSLIPIDEMIA

Abnormalities in lipid profiles are part of the increased atherogenic risk in obese children. The metabolic syndrome, common in obese children, is associated with the dyslipidemia triad (triglycerides >150 mg/dL, HDL cholesterol <40 mg/dL, LDL >130 mg/dL) (47).

In obese children 4 to 15 years of age, 45% had blood pressure above the 95th percentile for age and gender, 36% had increased insulin resistance defined as homeostasis model assessment (HOMA) greater than 4, 32% had hypertriglyceridemia, 13% had LDL higher than 150 mg/dL, and 5% had HDL cholesterol lower than 35 mg/dL (46). In a study of 13- to 16-year-olds, total cholesterol was correlated with BMI (48).

LDL cholesterol levels below 100 mg/dL are considered optimal. In children and adolescents, the criteria in Table 7.6 are used to determine elevated lipid levels (49).

State of the Problem

Excess LDL cholesterol can collect in the intima of the arterial wall. As LDL accumulates, the lipids undergo oxidation. Endothelial cells react to these changes by secreting cytokines, which attract monocytes to the intima. Monocytes then mature to active macrophages, which ingest the LDL particles. T cells also respond and, together with the LDL-containing macrophages, form a fatty streak (50).

As the inflammatory process progresses, smooth muscle cells of the media migrate to the top of the intima, producing a fibrous covering over the plaque. As

TABLE 7.5. *Classification of hypertension in children and adolescents, with measurement frequency and therapy recommendations*

	SBP or DBP percentile[a]	Frequency of BP measurement	Therapeutic lifestyle changes	Pharmacologic therapy
Normal	<90th	Recheck at next scheduled physical examination	Encourage healthy diet, sleep, and physical activity	—
Prehypertension	90th to <95th or if BP exceeds 120/80 even if <90th percentile up to <95th percentile[b]	Recheck in 6 mo	Weight-management counseling if overweight; introduce physical activity and diet management[c]	None unless compelling indications such as chronic kidney disease, diabetes mellitus, heart failure, or LVH exist
Stage 1 hypertension	95th–99th percentile plus 5 mm Hg	Recheck in 1–2 wk or sooner if the patient is symptomatic; if persistently elevated on 2 additional occasions, evaluate or refer to source of care within 1 mo	Weight-management counseling if overweight; introduce physical activity and diet management	Initiate therapy based on indications in Table 7.4 or if compelling indications (as shown above) exist
Stage 2 hypertension	>99th percentile plus 5 mm Hg	Evaluate or refer to source of care within 1 wk or immediately if the patient is symptomatic	Weight-management counseling if overweight; introduce physical activity and diet management	Initiate therapy[d]

BP, blood pressure; SBP, systolic blood pressure; DBP, diastolic blood pressure; LVH, left ventricular hypertrophy.

[a] For gender, age, and height measured on at least three separate occasions; if systolic and diastolic categories are different, categorize by the higher value.

[b] This occurs typically at 12 years old for SBP and at 16 years old for DBP.

[c] Parents and children trying to modify the eating plan to the Dietary Approaches to Stop Hypertension Study eating plan could benefit from consultation with a registered or licensed nutritionist to get them started.

[d] More than one drug may be required.

Reprinted with permission from National High Blood Pressure Education Program Working Group on High Blood Pressure in Children and Adolescents. The fourth report on the diagnosis, evaluation, and treatment of high blood pressure in children and adolescents. *Pediatrics.* 2004; 114:555–576.

inflammation continues or flares, the plaque can weaken and break open, causing a clot to form over the break and resulting in a heart attack or stroke (50).

Coronary artery calcification correlates with increased BMI in childhood and with increased blood pressure and decreased HDL cholesterol levels. Coronary risk

TABLE 7.6. *Criteria for determining elevated lipid levels*

	Low	Normal	High
Total cholesterol	<170 mg/dL	170–199 mg/dL	>200 mg/dL
HDL cholesterol	>40 mg/dL		<40 mg/dL
LDL cholesterol	<100 mg/dL	100–129 mg/dL	>130 mg/dL
Triglycerides	<200 mg/dL		>200 mg/dL

Reprinted with permission from Gidding SS, Dennison BA, Birch LL, Daniels SR, Gilman MW, Lichtenstein AH, Rattay KT, Steinberger J, Stettler N, Van Horn L; American Heart Association. American Heart Association Dietary Recommendations for Children and Adolescents: a guide for practitioners. *Pediatrics.* 2006;117:544–549.

factors in childhood and adolescence are associated with development of coronary artery calcification in young adult life (51).

Definitions

- **C-reactive protein (CRP)**—An acute phase protein and marker for systemic inflammation that has been associated with risk of coronary heart disease in adults (52).
- **Interleukin-6**—A proinflammatory cytokine expressed by adipose tissue that stimulates the production of CRP in the liver.

Treatment

Lifestyle changes aimed at improvement in nutrition, activity, and weight loss are the first steps in treating an obese child or adolescent with borderline or abnormal lipid levels (Table 7.7).

Weight loss is effective; a decrease in SDS-BMI of 0.5 or more over a year was associated with a significant lowering of systolic and diastolic blood pressure, LDL serum cholesterol, triglycerides, and insulin resistance and an increase in HDL cholesterol. LDL cholesterol decreased by a mean of 28 mg/dL, and triglycerides decreased by a mean of 82 mg/dL; HDL increased by a mean of 9 mg/dL and HOMA of insulin resistance decreased by a mean of 0.6 (46).

TABLE 7.7. *American Heart Association recommended pattern of nutrition and activity for cardiovascular health in all children and adolescents older than 2 years of age*

Eat foods low in saturated fat (<10% of calories/day), cholesterol (<300 mg/dL), trans fatty acids.
Include a variety of fruits, vegetables, whole grains, dairy products, and lean protein sources in the daily nutrition plan.
Match energy intake with energy needs for normal growth and development.
Limit intake of salt and sugar.
Passive and active cigarette smoking should be discouraged.
Physical activity for children and adolescents should be fun.
Children and adolescents should have 60 minutes of physical activity daily.

Reprinted with permission from Mahoney LT, Burns TL, Stanford W, et al. Coronary risk factors measured in childhood and young adult life are associated with coronary artery calcification in young adults: the Muscatine Study. *J Am Coll Cardiol.* 1996;27:277–284.

TABLE 7.8. *Other risk factors that contribute to earlier onset of coronary heart disease*

Family history of premature coronary heart disease, cerebrovascular disease, or occlusive
  peripheral vascular disease (definite onset before the age of 55 y in siblings, parent, or
  sibling of parent)
Cigarette smoking
Elevated blood pressure
Low HDL-cholesterol concentration (<35 mg/dL)
Obesity (≥95th BMI)
Diabetes mellitus
Physical inactivity

HDL, high-density lipoprotein; BMI, body mass index.
Reprinted with permission from Libby P. Vascular biology of atherosclerosis: overview and
state of the art. *Am J Cardiol.* 2003;91(3A):3A–6A.

The American Academy of Pediatrics statement "Cholesterol in Childhood" recommends that drug therapy be considered in children older than 10 years whose LDL cholesterol remains higher than 190 mg/dL after an adequate trial of dietary therapy (6–12 months). Pharmacologic treatment can also be considered if a child has an LDL cholesterol level that remains higher than 160 mg/dL, with two additional major risk factors (53) (Table 7.8).

The decision to initiate pharmacologic therapy should include careful consideration of both risk and protective factors, the latter including negative family history, female gender, and high HDL cholesterol (54). Cholestyramine, a bile acid binding resin, is approved for use in children. Absorption of medications may be affected, some of which include anticoagulants, digitalis, diuretics, penicillin G, phenylbutazone, propranolol, tetracycline, thyroid hormone, and vancomycin. Medical conditions that can be worsened by the use of cholestyramine include bleeding problems, constipation, gallstones, hemorrhoids, ulcers, hypothyroidism, renal disease, and phenylketonuria (55). Gastrointestinal side effects, including constipation, flatulence, and bloating, are common; fat-soluble vitamin malabsorption is a concern. Cholestyramine is contraindicated when triglyceride levels are higher than 400 mg/dL (54).

Triglyceride elevations are common in obese children, often associated with insulin resistance. A dietary plan should be the first course of treatment, focusing on decreasing the intake of simple sugars. If fasting levels of triglycerides are persistently elevated, evaluation for diabetes, thyroid disease, renal disease, and alcohol abuse is warranted (56). Fish oil (omega-3 fatty acids) can be used to treat hypertriglyceridemia (>500–700 mg/dL), usually at a dose of 2 g/day. Contact sports may be restricted because of an increased risk of bleeding (54). Specific pharmacologic treatment may be initiated at triglyceride levels higher than 400 mg/dL to protect against postprandial triglyceridemia of 1,000 mg/dL or greater, which may be associated with pancreatitis (54). Lovastatin (57), pravastatin (58), simvastatin (59), and atorvastatin (60), 3-hydroxy-3-methyl-glutaryl-CoA reductase (HMG-CoA reductase) inhibitors, have been studied in randomized trials of up to 48 weeks in the pediatric population. No long-term studies have been completed and these drugs are *not approved in pregnancy.* In one study of postmenarchal girls with familial hypercholesterolemia enrolled for 24 weeks, lovastatin treatment reduced LDL cholesterol by

23% to 25%, depending on dose (61). (Further discussion of pharmacotherapy for hyperlipidemia is found in Chapter 8, pp. 96–97.)

LEFT VENTRICULAR HYPERTROPHY

State of the Problem

> Left ventricular hypertrophy is the most prominent evidence of target end-organ damage from hypertension.

Etiology

Left ventricular hypertrophy is caused by hypertension in children and adolescents and has been reported in up to one third of children with mild, untreated hypertension (36).

Increased left ventricular mass is an independent predictor of coronary artery disease, stroke, and sudden death in adults. A left ventricular mass index of greater than 51 $g/m^{2.7}$ has been associated with a more than 3 times greater than normal risk of cardiovascular disease in adults (62). Left ventricular hypertrophy has been related to overweight in children. Lean body mass, fat mass, and systolic blood pressure have been shown to be independently associated with left ventricular mass in children and adolescents (63). In a study of 130 patients (6–23 years old) followed up in a hypertension clinic for at least 2 years, 8% had a left ventricular mass index greater than 51 $g/m^{2.7}$ (64).

Evaluation

Children and adolescents with hypertension should have an echocardiogram to determine if they have left ventricular hypertrophy. Left ventricular mass is calculated from measurements of intraventricular septal thickness, left ventricular end-diastolic dimension, and left ventricular posterior wall thickness (65).

Treatment

Weight loss has been shown to decrease left ventricular mass and blood pressure in children (66,67).

CARDIOMYOPATHY OF OBESITY

State of the Problem

> Cardiomyopathy of obesity is end-organ failure due to interacting effects of obesity on the heart.

Excessive obesity leads to an increase in blood volume and cardiac output caused by greater stroke volume. This increase in cardiac output leads to left ventricular dilation with increasing wall stress and resultant hypertrophy. When hypertrophy does not keep pace with ventricular dilation, wall stress becomes greater and systolic dysfunction may occur, resulting in left ventricular failure. Left ventricular failure can progress to pulmonary hypertension. If sleep apnea is also present, right ventricular failure may occur (68). In morbidly obese adults, increased blood flow and volume and impaired left ventricular compliance caused by left ventricular hypertrophy can predispose to diastolic dysfunction. The degree of dysfunction is affected by the duration of obesity (68). Obstructive sleep apnea has also been associated with left ventricular hypertrophy, diastolic dysfunction, and decrease in the nitric oxide–dependent dilatory capacity of the arterial wall (69).

Clinical Manifestations

In adults, signs and symptoms of obesity-related cardiomyopathy have been found in about 10% of patients whose BMI is greater than 40 kg/m^2, most of whom have been obese for more than 10 years (70). Clinical signs include the following (68):

- Progressive dyspnea on exertion
- Orthopnea
- Paroxysmal nocturnal dyspnea
- Lower extremity edema (68)

Cardiomegaly can be seen on chest radiograph (Fig. 7.1). In a study of obese children, mean left ventricular size, posterior wall thickness, and left ventricular mass were significantly greater than in normal weight children (71).

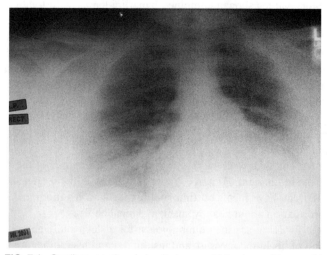

FIG. 7.1. Cardiomyopathy of obesity in a morbidly obese 17-year-old.

Treatment

Treatment of cardiac failure is primary, with long-term treatment focused on weight loss.

Case

Initial Presentation

BJ is a 17-year-old African American young man who comes to your office complaining of fatigue and worrying about his physical endurance. His weight is 146.6 kg (>95th percentile) and his height is 167.4 cm (10th percentile), with a BMI of 52.3 (>95th percentile). He says that he never really feels hungry, but his mother, who is with him, says that his portions are large. He has tried cutting back on eating and increasing his exercise but "nothing has worked." He is living with his mother and younger brother, neither of whom have a problem with weight. His father is not obese.

His dietary pattern is random, with frequent snacking, high consumption of sugar-containing beverages, and eating in his room. He has about 6 to 8 hours of combined computer and television time per day. He has recently tried a summer intramural basketball league, and his performance prompted his concerns about endurance. He is a senior, and his grades are good.

His family history is positive for hypertension, high cholesterol, and cardiovascular disease in his first- and second-degree relatives and for diabetes in the extended family.

His review of systems is positive for inhaler use for exercise asthma, snoring, orthopnea, and daytime tiredness.

On physical examination, his blood pressure is 138/72 mm Hg (systolic >95th percentile). He has acanthosis nigricans and a waist circumference of 132 cm.

His laboratory values show a combined hyperlipidemia, with total cholesterol of 191 mg/dL, triglycerides of 190 mg/dL, LDL cholesterol of 122 mg/dL, and HDL of 31 mg/dL. His fasting insulin is mildly elevated at 30 U/mL. Fasting blood glucose and liver function studies are normal. His metabolic panel is also normal.

You outline the medical problems, which include possible sleep apnea, metabolic syndrome, elevated blood pressure, and morbid obesity with probable significant deconditioning.

You link these comorbidities with his weight and assess BJ's and the family's interest in beginning to make lifestyle change. His mother is supportive of change to help him, and BJ wants to lose weight.

The first step you take with the family is to suggest eliminating the sugared beverages. Both the mother and BJ agree. You also work with them on a structured eating plan, so BJ can have meals on time and dinner with his mom and brother. You give them information about healthy snack and meal choices.

You arrange for BJ to see the pulmonologist for a sleep study and plan for ongoing monitoring of his blood pressure and insulin. BJ and his mother are scheduled to return in 4 weeks.

Second Visit

BJ and his mother are in your office. His weight is 143.6 kg, his height is 167.4 cm, and his BMI is 50.88. His blood pressure is 142/88 mm Hg. He has switched to diet drinks, started eating breakfast, and decreased his intake of cheese. BJ reports he is feeling slightly less hungry and a little more energetic. He is on the schedule for a sleep study. You reinforce his progress, set a goal of daily walking, and ask him to return in 1 month.

Third Visit

On the third visit, BJ's weight is 142.5 kg, down 4.1 kg from his initial visit. His blood pressure is 128/78 mm Hg; you put him on Vasotec 5 mg/day to start treatment and order an echocardiogram. He has been doing "a little walking." His sleep study was completed and showed significant sleep apnea. Bilevel airway pressure (BiPAP) was recommended, and so far he refuses to use it. You discuss the implications of sleep apnea with him, including the effect on blood pressure, and he says he will "try." You reschedule an appointment for 2 months because of the mother's concern that BJ will miss school.

Fourth Visit

BJ returns after 2 months. His weight is 137.1 kg, which makes a total weight loss of 9.5 kg. His blood pressure is 126/72 mm Hg. He has tried his BiPAP a few nights and reports that he feels better after using it but is still having trouble with consistent use. He has begun to play flag football with his friends and is feeling more optimistic about his performance. You encourage continued diet and activity changes.

Fifth Visit

Two months later, BJ returns with a weight of 132.8 kg, down 13.8 kg total. Laboratory studies show a total cholesterol of 172 mg/dL, triglycerides of 111 mg/dL, and insulin of 6.8 µU/mL. He is happier with himself, is doing well in school, and has begun to wear his BiPAP almost all the time.

REFERENCES

1. World Health Organization. Cardiovascular Disease Facts. http://www.who.int/dietphysicalactivity/publications/facts/cvd/en/ (accessed 5/1/06).
2. Relationship of atherosclerosis in young men to serum lipoprotein cholesterol concentrations and smoking: a preliminary report from the Pathobiological Determinants of Atherosclerosis in Youth (PDAY) Research Group. *JAMA.* 1990;264:3018–3024.
3. Berenson GS, Srinivasan SR, Bao W, Newman WP 3rd, Tracy RE, Wattigney WA. Association between multiple cardiovascular risk factors and atherosclerosis in children and young adults. The Bogalusa Heart Study. *N Engl J Med.* 1998;338:1650–1656.
4. Daniels SR, Arnett DK, Eckel RH, Gidding SS, Hayman LL, Kumanyika S, Robinson TN, Scott BJ, St Jeor S, Williams CL. Overweight in children and adolescents: pathophysiology, consequences, prevention and treatment. *Circulation.* 2005;111:1999–2012.

5. Freedman DS, Serdula MK, Srinivassan SR, Berenson GS. The relation of circumference and skinfolds to levels of lipids and insulin: the Bogalusa Heart Study. *Am J Clin Nutr.* 1999;69:308–317.

6. Ford ES. Galuska DA, Gillespie C, Will JC, Giles WH, Dietz WH. C reactive protein and body mass index in children findings of the Third National Health and Nutrition Examination Survey 1988-1994. *J Pediatr.* 2001;138:486–492.

7. Pilz S, Horejsi R, Moller R, Almer G, Scharnagl H, Stojakovic T, Dimitrova R, Weihrauch G, Borkenstein M, Maerz W, Schauenstein K, Mangge H. Early atherosclerosis in obese juveniles is associated with low serum levels of adiponectin. *J Clin Endocrinol Metab.* 2005;90:4792–4796.

8. Estelles A, Dalmau J, Falco C, Berbel O, Castello R, Espana F, Aznar J. Plasma PA-1 levels in obese children: effect of weight loss and influence of PAI-1 promoter 4G/5G genotype. *Thromb Haemost.* 2001;86:647–652.

9. Gallistl S, Sudi K, Mangge H, Erwa W, Borkenstein M. Insulin is an independent correlate of plasma homocysteine levels in obese children and adolescents. *Diabetes Care.* 2000;23:1348–1352.

10. Freedman DS, Dietz WH, Srinivasan SR, Berenson GS. The relation of overweight to cardiovascular risk factors among children and adolescents: the Bogalusa Heart Study. *Pediatrics.* 1999;103(6 Pt 1): 1175–1182.

11. Janssen I, Katzmarzyk PT, Srinivasan SR, Chen W, Malina RM, Bouchard C, Berenson GS. Combined influence of body mass index and waist circumference on coronary artery disease risk factors among children and adolescents. *Pediatrics.* 2005;115:1623–1630.

12. Gidding SS, Nehgme R, Heise C, Muscar C, Linton A, Hassink S. Severe obesity associated with cardiovascular deconditioning, high prevalence of cardiovascular risk factors, diabetes mellitus/hyperinsulinemia, and respiratory compromise. *J Pediatr.* 2004;144:766–769.

13. Visser M, Bouter LM, McQuillan GM, Wener MH, Harris TB. Low grade systemic inflammation in overweight children. *Pediatrics.* 2001;107(1):e 13.

14. Isasi CR, Deckelbaum RJ, Tracy RP, Starc TJ, Berglund L, Shea S. Physical fitness and C reactive protein level in children and young adults: The Columbia University Bio Markers Study. *Pediatrics.* 2003;111:332–338.

15. Cohen MS. Fetal and childhood onset of adult cardiovascular disease. *Pediatr Clin North Am.* 2004;51:1697–1719.

16. Leeson CP, Whincup PH, Cook DG, Donald AE, Papacosta O, Lucas A, Deanfield JE. Flow mediated dilation in 9 to 11 year old children: the influence of intrauterine and childhood factors. *Circulation.* 1997;96:2233–2238.

17. Woo KS, Chook P, Yu CW, Sung RY, Qiao M, Leung SS, Lam CW, Metreweli C, Celermajer DS. Overweight in children is associated with arterial endothelial dysfunction and intima-media thickening. *Int J Obes Relat Metab Disord.* 2004;28:1–6.

18. Barker DJ. The intrauterine origins of cardiovascular disease. *Acta Paediatr Suppl.* 1993;82(Suppl 391):93–99.

19. Hales CN, Barker DJ, Clark PM, Cox LJ, Fall C, Osmond C, Winter PD. Fetal and infant growth and impaired glucose tolerance at age 64. *BMJ.* 1991;303:1019–1022.

20. Martyn CN, Barker DJ, Osmond C. Mothers pelvic size, fetal growth, and death from stroke and coronary heart disease in men in the UK. *Lancet.* 1996;348:1264–1268.

21. Barker DJ, Bull AR, Osmond C, Simmonds SJ. Fetal and placental size and risk of hypertension in adult life. *BMJ.* 1990;301:259–262.

22. Barker DJ, Hales CN, Fall CH, Osmond C, Phipps K, Clark PM. Type 2 (non insulin dependent) diabetes mellitus, hypertension and hyperlipidemia (syndrome X): relation to reduced fetal growth. *Diabetologia.* 1993;36:62–67.

23. Ong KK, Dunger DB. Perinatal growth failure: the road to obesity insulin resistance and cardiovascular disease in adults. *Best Pract Res Clin Endocrinol Metab.* 2002;16:191–207.

24. Forsen T, Eriksson J, Tuomilehto J, Reunanen A, Osmond C, Barker D. The fetal and childhood growth of person who develop type 2 diabetes. *Ann Intern Med.* 2000;133:176–182.

25. Phillips DI, Walker BR, Reynolds RM, Flanagan DE, Wood PJ, Osmond C, Barker DJ, Whorwood CB. Low birth weight predicts elevated plasma cortisol concentrations in adults from 3 populations. *Hypertension.* 2000;35:1301–1306.

26. Phillips DI, Barker DJ, Fall CH, Seckl JR, Whorwood CB, Wood PJ, Walker BR. Elevated plasma cortisol concentrations: a link between low birth weight and the insulin resistance syndrome? *J Clin Endocrinol Metab.* 1998;83:757–760.

27. World Health Report 2002. Reducing risks, promoting healthy life. http://www.who.int/whr/2002/en/ p. 69 (accessed 5/2/06).

28. Falkner B, Kushner H, Onesti G, Angelakos ET. Cardiovascular characteristics in adolescents who develop essential hypertension. *Hypertension.* 198;13:521–527.
29. Bao W, Threefoot SA, Srinivasan SR, Berenson GS. Essential hypertension predicted by tracking of elevated blood pressure from childhood to adulthood: the Bogalusa Heart Study. *Am J Hypertens.* 1995;8:657–665.
30. Sorof JM, Lai D, Turner J, Poffenbarger T, Portman RJ. Overweight, ethnicity, and the prevalence of hypertension in school-aged children. *Pediatrics.* 2004;113(3 Pt 1):475–482.
31. Falkner B, Gidding SS, Ramirez-Garnica G, Wiltrout SA, West D, Rappaport EB. The relationship of body mass index and blood pressure in primary care pediatric patients. *J Pediatr.* 2006;148:195–200.
32. Portman RJ, McNiece KL, Swinford RD, Braun MC, Samuels JA. Pediatric hypertension: diagnosis, evaluation, management and treatment for the primary care physician. *Curr Probl Pediatr Adolesc Health Care.* 2005;35:262–294.
33. Kaufmann MA, Pargger H, Drop LJ. Oscillometric blood pressure measurement by different devices are not interchangeable. *Anesth Analg.* 1996;82:377–381.
34. Chobanian AV, Bakris GL, Black HR, Cushman WC, Green LA, Izzo JL Jr, Jones DW, Materson BJ, Oparil S, Wright JT JR, Roccella EJ; National Heart, Lung and Blood Institute Joint National Committee on Prevention, Detection, Evaluation and Treatment of High Blood Pressure. National Heart, Lung and Blood Institute; National High Blood Pressure Education Program Coordinating Committee. Seventh report of the Joint National Committee on Prevention, Detection, Evaluation and Treatment of High Blood Pressure. *Hypertension.* 2003;42:1206–1253.
35. Freedman, DS, Khan LK, Dietz WH, Srinivasan SR, Berenson GS. Relationship of childhood obesity to coronary heart disease risk factors in adulthood: The Bogalusa Heart Study. *Pediatrics.* 2001;108:712–718.
36. National High Blood Pressure Education Program Working Group on High Blood Pressure in Children and Adolescents. The fourth report on the diagnosis, evaluation and treatment of high blood pressure in children and adolescents. *Pediatrics.* 2004;114(2 Suppl):555–576.
37. Davis PH, Dawson JD, Riley WA, Lauer RM. Carotid intimal medial thickness is related to cardiovascular risk factors measured from childhood through middle age: the Muscatine Study. *Circulation.* 2001;104:2815–2819.
38. Arnett DK, Glasser SP, McVeigh G, Prineas R, Finklestein S, Donahue R, Cohn JN, Sinaiko A. Blood pressure and arterial compliance in young adults: the Minnesota Children's Blood Pressure study. *Am J Hypertens.* 2001;14:200–205.
39. DeFronzo RA. The effect of insulin on renal sodium metabolism A review with clinical implications. *Diabetologia.* 1981;21:165–171.
40. Antic V, Dulloo A, Montani JP. Multiple mechanisms involved in obesity-induced hypertension. *Heart Lung Circ.* 2003;12(2):84–93.
41. Hall JE, Brands MW, Henegar JR. Mechanisms of hypertension and kidney disease in obesity. *Ann N Y Acad Sci.* 1999;892:91–107.
42. Ribeiro MM, Silva AG, Santos NS, Guazzelle I, Matos LN, Trombetta IC, Halpern A, Negrao CE, Villares SM. Diet and exercise training restore blood pressure and vasodilatory responses during physiological maneuvers in obese children. *Circulation.* 2005;111:1915–1923.
43. Haynes WG. Role of leptin in obesity-related hypertension. *Exp Physiol.* 2005;90:683–688.
44. Watkins LL, Sherwood A, Feinglos M, Hinderliter A, Babyak M, Gullette E, Waugh R, Blumenthal JA. Effects of exercise and weight loss on cardiac risk factors associated with syndrome X. *Arch Intern Med.* 2003;163:1889–1895.
45. Stern JS, Hirsch J, Blair SN, Foreyt JP, Frank A, Kumanyika SK, Madans JH, Marlatt GA, St Jeor ST, Stunkard AJ. Weighing the options—criteria for evaluating weight management programs. The committee to develop criteria for evaluating the outcomes of approaches to prevent and treat obesity. *Obes Res.* 1995;3:591–604.
46. Reinehr T, Andler W. Changes in the atherogenic risk factor profile according to degree of weight loss. *Arch Dis Child.* 2004;89:419–420.
47. Sinaiko AR, Donahue RP, Jacobs DR, Prineas RJ. Relation of weight and rate of increase in weight during childhood and adolescence to body size, blood pressure, fasting insulin, and lipids in young adults. The Minneapolis Children's Blood Pressure Study. *Circulation.* 1999;99:1471–1476.
48. Owen CG, Whincup PH, Odoki K, Gilg JA, Cook DG. Birth weight and blood cholesterol level: a study in adolescents and systematic review. *Pediatrics.* 2003;111(5 Pt 1):1081–1089.
49. Gidding SS, Dennison BA, Birch LL, Daniels SR, Gilman MW, Lichtenstein AH, Rattay KT, Steinberger J, Stettler N, Van Horn L; American Heart Association. American Heart Association Dietary

Recommendations for Children and Adolescents: a guide for practitioners. *Pediatrics*. 2006;117: 544–549.

50. Libby P. Vascular biology of atherosclerosis; overview and state of the art. *Am J Cardiol*. 2003; 91(3A):3A–6A.

51. Mahoney LT, Burns TL, Stanford W, Thompson BH, Witt JD, Rost CA, Lauer RM. Coronary risk factors measured in childhood and young adult life are associated with coronary artery calcification in young adults: the Muscatine Study. *J Am Coll Cardiol*. 1996;27:277–284.

52. Lowe GD. Circulating inflammatory markers and risks of cardiovascular and non-cardiovascular disease. *J Thromb Haemost*. 2005;3:1618–1627.

53. American Academy of Pediatrics. Cholesterol in Childhood Committee on Nutrition. *Pediatrics*. 1998;101:141–147.

54. Gidding SS. Cardiovascular risk factors in adolescents. *Curr Treat Options Cardiovasc Med*. 2006;8.

55. Medline plus. http://www.nlm.nih.gov/medlineplus/druginfo/uspdi/202137.html (accessed 5/3/06).

56. Kavey RE, Daniels SR, Lauer RM, Atkins DL, Hayman LL, Taubert K; American Heart Association. American Heart Association guideline for primary prevention of atherosclerotic cardiovascular disease beginning childhood. *Circulation*. 2003;107:1562–1566.

57. Stein EA, Illingworth DR, Kwiterovich PO Jr, Liacouras CA Siimes MA, Jacobson MS, Brewster TG, Hopkins P, Davidson M, Graham K, Arensman F, Knopp RH, DuJovne C, Williams CL, Isaachsohn JL, Jacobsen CA, Laskarzewski PM. Ames S, Gormley GJ. Efficacy and safety of lovastatin in adolescent males with heterozygous familial hypercholesterolemia: a randomized controlled trial. *JAMA*. 1999;281:137–144.

58. Wiegman A, Hutten BA, deGroot E, Rodenburg J, Bakker HD, Buller HR, Sijbrands EJ, Kastelein JJ. Efficacy and safety of statin therapy in children with familial hypercholesterolemia a randomized controlled trial. *JAMA*. 2004;292:331–337.

59. deJongh S, Ose L, Szamosi T, Gagne C, Lambert M, Scott R, Perron P, Dobbelaere D, Saborio M, Tuohy MB, Stepanavage M, Sapre A, Gumbiner B, Mercuri M, van Trotsenburg AS, Bakker HD, Kastelein JJ; Simvastatin in Children Study Group. Efficacy and safety of statin therapy in children with familial hypercholesterolemia: a randomized, double blind, placebo controlled trial with Simvastatin. *Circulation*. 2002;106:2231–2237.

60. McCrindle BW, Ose L, Marais AD. Efficacy and safety of atorvastatin in children and adolescents with familial hypercholesterolemia or severe hyperlipidemia: a multicenter, randomized placebo-controlled trial. *J Pediatr*. 2003;439:74–80.

61. Clauss SB, Holmes KW, Hopkins P, Stein E, Cho M, Tate A, Johnson-Levonas AO, Kwiterovich PO. Efficacy in and safety of lovastatin therapy in adolescent girls with heterozygous familial hypercholesterolemia. *Pediatrics*. 2005;116:682–688.

62. de Simone G, Devereux RB, Daniels SR, Koren MJ, Meyer RA, Laragh JH. Effect of growth on variability of left ventricular mass: assessment of allometric signals in adults and children and their capacity to predict cardiovascular risk. *J Am Coll Cardiol*. 1995;25:1056–1062.

63. Daniels SR, Kimball TR, Morrison JA, Khoury P, Witt S, Meyer RA. Effect of lean body mass, fat mass, blood pressure, and sexual maturation on left ventricular mass in children and adolescents. Statistical, biological and clinical significance. *Circulation*. 1995;92:3249–3254.

64. Daniels SR, Loggie JM, Khoury P, Kimball TR. Left ventricular geometry and severe left ventricular hypertrophy in children and adolescents with essential hypertension. *Circulation*. 1998;97: 1907–1911.

65. de Simone G, Daniels SR, Devereux RB, Meyer RA, Roman MJ, de Divitiis O, Alderman MH. Left ventricular mass and heart size in normotensive children and adults: assessment of allometric relations and impact of overweight. *J Am Coll Cardiol*. 1992;20:1251–1260.

66. Rocchini AP, Katch V, Anderson J, Hinderliter J, Becque D, Martin M, Marks C. Blood pressure in obese adolescents: effect of weight loss. *Pediatrics*. 1988;82:16–23.

67. MacMahon SW, Wilcken DEL, Macdonald GJ. The effect of weight reduction on left ventricular mass: a randomized controlled trial in young overweight hypertensive patients. *N Engl J Med*. 1986;314:334–339.

68. Alpert MA. Obesity cardiomyopathy: pathophysiology and evolution of the clinical syndrome. *Am J Med Sci*. 2001;321:225–236.

69. Kraiczi H, Caidahl K, Samuelsson A, Peker Y, Hedner J. Impairment of vascular endothelial function and left ventricular filling association with the severity of apnea induced hypoxemia during sleep. *Chest*. 2001;119:1085–1091.

70. Alexander JK. Obesity and the heart. *Curr Prob Cardiol*. 1980;5(3):6–41.

71. Yoshinaga M, Yuasa Y, Hatano H, Kono Y, Nomura Y, Oku S, Nakamura M, Kanekura S, Otsubo K, Akiba S, et al. Effect of total adipose weight and systemic hypertension of left ventricular mass in children. *Am J Cardiol*. 1995;76:785–787.

8

Insulin Resistance, the Metabolic Syndrome, and Type 2 Diabetes

OVERVIEW

A major metabolic implication of the obesity epidemic is the rapid rise in the number of children and adolescents in whom type 2 diabetes is diagnosed or is developing. Type 2 diabetes evolves over time along a continuum of metabolic derangement beginning with insulin resistance.

Obesity in childhood and adolescence has been shown to increase the risk of insulin resistance (1). Insulin resistance has been linked to hypertension, dyslipidemia, polycystic ovarian syndrome (PCOS), and nonalcoholic steatohepatitis (NASH) in children and adolescents with obesity (2). Insulin resistance is a signal feature in the metabolic syndrome, a phenotype first defined by Reaven (3) as "syndrome X." The metabolic syndrome is defined as obesity, elevated blood pressure, elevated triglyceride, decreased HDL cholesterol levels, and impaired glucose tolerance (IGT). Specific definitions vary, and long-term studies are needed to establish the nature of the link between these risk factors and later morbidity (4–6).

As a result of the obesity-driven rise in insulin resistance, the incidence of IGT is increased in obese children. As insulin resistance increases, the first-phase insulin response is lost, resulting in IGT. In one study, 25% of children and 21% of adolescents presenting to an obesity clinic for treatment had IGT, and 4% of adolescents were newly diagnosed with diabetes (7). In these patients, insulin and C-peptide levels were elevated and IGT was associated with insulin resistance, the first phase of the evolution of type 2 diabetes.

State of the Problem

The increase of type 2 diabetes in adults has paralleled the rising prevalence of obesity. Diabetes now affects 7.7% of the adult American population, or 16 million individuals. Adults with a body mass index (BMI) greater than 40 are 7.4 times more likely to develop diabetes than their normal weight counterparts (8). Type 2 diabetes may range from a predominantly insulin-resistant form treatable with oral agents to a predominantly secretory defect requiring insulin treatment (9).

Paralleling this increase in adults, children and adolescents are also being affected, and the occurrence of type 2 diabetes in childhood is no longer a rarity. Driven by the rise in obesity, type 2 diabetes, in some series (10), comprises 30% of all newly diagnosed cases of diabetes in 10- to 20-year-old patients. Increases in incidence among Native American, African American, and Hispanic children have been particularly striking in the United States (11).

This escalating incidence has been mirrored across the globe, particularly in populations shifting from relative undernutrition to overnutrition (12). In the 1970s and 1980s, type 2 diabetes in children was reported in the Native American (1979) and Canadian First Nation (1984) populations. By the mid 1990s ethnic minorities (African Americans, Hispanic Americans) were experiencing rapidly rising rates of disease, as were children in Japan and Asian populations, and by 2000 cases were emerging in Europe (13).

The onset of diabetes in childhood and adolescence substantially increases the risk of significant morbidity and mortality from retinopathy, nephropathy, neuropathy, and cardiovascular disease at a younger age. Diabetes-associated microvascular and macrovascular complications evolve based on duration of disease and extent of hyperglycemia. Early signs of microvascular change, dyslipidemia, and hypertension are already present at diagnosis in some populations of children (14).

Definitions

- **Insulin resistance**—An impaired ability of plasma insulin at usual concentrations to adequately promote peripheral glucose disposal, suppress hepatic glucose, and inhibit very low density lipoprotein output (8).
- **Prediabetes**—A period of either elevated fasting glucose levels or IGT occurring before the development of type 2 diabetes (15). Prediabetes is defined as fasting glucose greater than or equal to 100 mg/dL and less than 126 mg/dL, or a 2-hour post–glucose load plasma glucose level greater than or equal to 140 mg/dL and less than 200 mg/dL (16).
- **GLUT4**—A glucose transporter isoform that is the major insulin-responsive transporter. It is located in striated muscle and adipose tissue. GLUT4 transporter proteins are enclosed in intracellular storage vesicles that respond to rising postprandial glucose levels by migrating to the plasma membrane, allowing tissues to respond to fluctuations in circulating insulin levels (17).

Etiology

The evolution of type 2 diabetes involves the development of both insulin resistance and beta cell failure and progresses over time with a gradual decline in beta cell function (18). First-phase insulin secretion is initially lost, with an inability of endogenous insulin secretion to compensate for the evolving insulin resistance (19). The cause of insulin resistance, insulin resistance syndrome, and type 2 diabetes is multifactorial.

Type 2 diabetes develops in the setting of genetic predisposition and a permissive nutritional and activity environment. The addition of obesity to genetic risk factors is undoubtedly fueling the current rise in the incidence of type 2 diabetes. Further evidence for the influence of genetics on diabetes risk comes from the wide variation of diabetes prevalence in different ethnic groups when all share similar environments (20).

Obesity in adults can modulate insulin sensitivity secondary to an increase in visceral fat (21). Visceral fat correlates with insulin levels in children (22). Children with greater central adiposity develop metabolic syndrome more frequently than children with peripheral body fat distribution (23). In this same study, waist circumference correlated more strongly to metabolic syndrome than either BMI or skin fold thickness (23). In a study of Hispanic children with increased waist-to-hip ratios, visceral fat measurements were positively correlated to both fasting insulin and acute insulin response to glucose. In the same study, visceral fat measurement was negatively related to insulin sensitivity (24).

Obese children and adolescents with IGT have increased intramyocellular lipid levels and visceral-to-subcutaneous-abdominal-fat ratios when compared with obese nonimpaired individuals (18). Intramyocellular accumulation of lipid causes abnormalities in insulin signaling (18, 25).

> The presence of high levels of triglycerides in muscle cells impairs glucose oxidation and insulin response (26).

In a study of obese children and adolescents, intramyocellular lipid and visceral-to-subcutaneous-fat ratio were positively related to the 2-hour plasma glucose level during an oral glucose tolerance test (OGTT) (18). Leptin, which is increased in obesity, may be involved in the regulation of insulin sensitivity and triglyceride levels (26).

Type 2 diabetes is more common in African American children than in white children. During hyperglycemic clamp studies in normal weight children, African American children exhibited higher insulin levels than did their white peers (27). The Bogalusa Heart Study showed increased insulin response to the oral glucose tolerance test in African American versus white children after adjusting for Tanner stage and weight (28).

Collectively, more than 600 genes, markers, and chromosomal regions have been associated or linked with human obesity phenotypes (29). Genetic and familial findings that relate to diabetes include the following:

• Individual genetic predispositions to type 2 diabetes exist; 75% to 100% of children and adults with type 2 diabetes have a first- or second-degree relative with type 2 diabetes (30).

- Insulin sensitivity in nondiabetic children from families with a history of type 2 diabetes has been found to be decreased by 20% (31).
- β-Adrenergic receptor subtypes have been associated with obesity and type 2 diabetes (32).
- In adults, the concordance rate of type 2 diabetes in monozygotic twins is approximately 90%, and the lifetime risk of type 2 diabetes in a first-degree relative is approximately 40% (33).

Interactions between shifts in energy balance and predisposition to insulin resistance and type 2 diabetes may occur. Such interactions may involve population risk, as when Neal (12) noted in 1962 that an unexpectedly high rate of type 2 diabetes was found in populations shifting from a history of relative undernutrition to overnutrition. He proposed that a "thrifty genotype" of energy conservation had developed to confer a survival advantage in these groups. This hypothesis may be true for several of the ethnic groups with high rates of type 2 diabetes, such as the Pima Indians.

Energy availability in the intrauterine environment may be another determinant of diabetes risk. Children who were infants of diabetic mothers were found to have increased rates of IGT as young as 2 to 5 years of age (34). Exposure to hyperinsulinemia and increased glucose *in utero* during pregnancy in a diabetic woman can result in macrosomia at birth and an increased risk of obesity, IGT in childhood, and future diabetes (35,36). In addition, infants of diabetic mothers who had a greater intake of breast milk from their mothers had a higher relative body weight at 2 years and a correlation of breast milk intake with postprandial glucose levels (37).The significance of this finding has yet to be determined.

Low birth weight has also been associated with increased rates of type 2 diabetes later in life (38).

> The "thrifty phenotype" hypothesis was advanced to propose that early exposure of the fetus to poor nutrition leads to permanent changes in insulin metabolism and body fat distribution (35).

Low birth weight has also been associated with increased central fat deposition in children (39) and higher rates of type 2 diabetes later in life (40). In a Finnish study, children who later developed type 2 diabetes had lower birth weight, lower weight at 1 year, and an early tendency to develop adiposity (41). These findings fit with animal models of prenatal growth restriction followed by postnatal ad lib feeding, which results in insulin resistance and diabetes (42).

The increase in insulin resistance during normal puberty may also enhance the risk of type 2 diabetes because the predominant defect in type 2 diabetes is peripheral resistance to the effects of insulin with a variable insulin secretory deficit (43). In one study, insulin-mediated glucose disposal was 30% lower in pubertal versus prepubertal children and young adults (44). This is thought to be due to the pubertal increase in growth hormone secretion (43). It is worth noting that African American children

TABLE 8.1. *Glucose tolerance test results*

- FPG <100 mg/dL (5.6 mmol/L) = normal fasting glucose
- FPG 100–125 mg/dL (5.6–6.9 mmol/L) = impaired fasting glucose (IFG)
- FPG ≥126 mg/dL (7.0 mmol/L) = provisional diagnosis of diabetes (the diagnosis must be confirmed, as described below)

The corresponding categories when the OGTT is used are the following:

- 2-hr post load glucose <140 mg/dL (7.8 mmol/L) = normal glucose tolerance
- 2-hr post load glucose 140–199 mg/dL (7.8–11.1 mmol/L) = impaired glucose tolerance (IGT)
- 2-hr post load glucose ≥200 mg/dL (11.1 mmol/L) = provisional diagnosis of diabetes (the diagnosis must be confirmed, as described below)

FPG, fasting plasma glucose; OGTT, oral glucose tolerance test.

Note that many individuals with IGT are euglycemic in their daily lives. Individuals with IFG or IGT may have normal or near normal glycosylated hemoglobin levels. Individuals with IGT often manifest hyperglycemia only when challenged with the oral glucose load used in the standardized OGTT (1,2).

Reprinted with permission from American Diabetes Association Position Statements Original Article Diagnosis and Classification of Diabetes Mellitus. *Diabetes Care.* 2005;28:S37–S42.

do not have the same level of compensatory increase in insulin secretion that white children do in response to high levels of growth hormone during puberty. This may explain their increased risk for type 2 diabetes during this phase of growth (14).

Clinical Manifestations

Impaired Glucose Tolerance and Impaired Fasting Glucose

Patients with impaired fasting glucose (IFG) and/or IGT are now referred to as having "prediabetes," indicating the relatively high risk for development of diabetes in these patients. IFG and IGT are associated with the metabolic syndrome, which includes obesity (especially abdominal or visceral obesity), dyslipidemia [of the high-triglyceride and/or low–high-density lipoprotein (HDL) type], and hypertension (45,46). IFG reference limits were decreased to greater than 100 mg/dL by the Expert Committee on Diagnosis and Classification of Diabetes Mellitus (46). However, the correlation between IFG and IGT is still not perfect, and the OGTT remains the defining test for IGT (47) (Table 8.1). With appropriate changes in lifestyle, progression from IGT to diabetes can be delayed or prevented (48).

Risk Factors

The current rise in the rates of type 2 diabetes can be thought of as the unmasking of underlying individual genetic susceptibility by social, behavioral, and environmental risk factors (14).

Risk factors for type 2 diabetes include the following:

- Ethnicity
- Obesity
- Puberty

- Positive family history
- Polycystic ovarian syndrome (PCOS)
- Acanthosis nigricans
- Decreased physical activity (49)
- Maternal diabetes
- Maternal gestational diabetes (50)

Acanthosis Nigricans

Acanthosis nigricans is associated with insulin resistance and hyperinsulinemia and features of the metabolic syndrome. Prevalence in the general population has been reported as follows:

- 13.3% in African American children
- 5.5% in Hispanic children
- 0.5% in white children (51)

Insulin Resistance

The American Heart Association (52) defines

- Normal fasting insulin in children as insulin <15 µU/mL (following a 12-hour fast)
- Borderline high fasting insulin as 15 to 20 µU/mL
- High fasting insulin as >20 µU/mL

TYPE 2 DIABETES

The presentation of type 2 diabetes can range from asymptomatic glycosuria to ketonuria or ketoacidosis with dehydration and weight loss (30). However, individuals with type 2 diabetes often present with obesity, glycosuria but no ketonuria, mild or absent polyuria and polydipsia, and little or no recent weight loss. Most will also have acanthosis nigricans (53). In one study, 25% of girls diagnosed with type 2 diabetes presented with vaginal candidiasis (54). Type 2 diabetes should be suspected in the presence of obesity-related comorbidities, such as acanthosis nigricans, hypertension, sleep apnea, PCOS, and NASH.

Recommendations by the American Diabetic Association (ADA) consensus panel of experts for screening for type 2 diabetes include any patient who has a BMI greater than the 85th percentile for age and gender and two of the following risk factors: (a) family history of type 2 diabetes in first- or second-degree relatives; (b) belonging to an ethnic group of African Americans, Hispanic Americans, American Indians, or Asians/South Pacific Islanders; and (c) having insulin resistance or conditions associated with insulin resistance such as PCOS, acanthosis nigricans, hypertension, or dyslipidemia. If the requirements for BMI and two other criteria are met, testing should start at age 10 years (or at onset of pubertal development if it occurs earlier than age 10) and be continued every 2 years. The expert panel also recommended that clinical judgment be used in testing any other patients believed to be at high risk for diabetes. Fasting plasma glucose is the preferred screen (9).

Diagnosis

The ADA diagnostic criteria for type 2 diabetes in children are listed in Table 8.2. Patients with type 2 diabetes can present with diabetic ketoacidosis, and there has also been a recent report of adolescents who presented with hyperglycemic hyperosmolar state (HHS) as the first recognized manifestation of type 2 diabetes. In several patients, this condition resulted in death. These patients had initial clinical symptoms that included the following:

- Vomiting
- Abdominal pain
- Dizziness
- Weakness
- Polyuria
- Polydipsia
- Weight loss
- Diarrhea

These patients presented acutely with what was thought to be diabetic ketoacidosis but was eventually recognized as HHS. The diagnostic criteria for HHS include a plasma glucose level of more than 600 mg/dL, serum carbon dioxide level of more than 15 mmol/L, small ketonuria, absent to low ketonemia, an effective serum osmolality of more than 320 mOsm/kg, and stupor or coma (55,56).

Along with diabetic ketoacidosis, HHS represents an acute emergency.

TABLE 8.2. *Criteria for the diagnosis of diabetes mellitus*

1. Symptoms of diabetes plus casual plasma glucose concentration ≥200 mg/dL (11.1 mmol/L). Casual is defined as any time of day without regard to time since the last meal. The classic symptoms of diabetes include polyuria, polydipsia, and unexplained weight loss.
   or
2. FPG ≥126 mg/dL (7.0 mmol/L). Fasting is defined as no caloric intake for at least 8 hr.
3. 2-hr post load glucose ≥200 mg/dL (11.1 mmol/L) during an OGTT. The test should be performed as described by WHO, using a glucose load containing the equivalent of 75 g anhydrous glucose dissolved in water.

In the absence of unequivocal hyperglycemia, these criteria should be confirmed by repeat testing on a different day. The third measure (OGTT) is not recommended for routine clinical use.

OGTT, oral glucose tolerance test; WHO, World Health Organization.
Reprinted with permission from American Diabetes Association Position Statements Original Article Diagnosis and Classification of Diabetes Mellitus. *Diabetes Care.* 2005;28:S37–S42.

Goals of Treatment

The goals of treatment for type 2 diabetes in children and adolescents are to achieve normal growth and development and include the following:

1. Physical well-being (15)
2. Weight loss or no further weight gain (30)
3. Continued normal linear growth (30)
4. Psychological well-being (15)
5. Long-term glycemic control (30,49)
   a. HgbA$_{1C}$ should be maintained at minimum less than 7%
   b. Lifestyle intervention (diet, exercise, and weight control) initially
   c. Pharmacotherapy if lifestyle change does not achieve glycemic control with metformin as initial therapy
   d. The addition of insulin if control is not achieved with metformin and lifestyle change (15)
6. Control of hypertension and hyperlipidemia (30)

Prevention of Microvascular and Macrovascular Complications of Diabetes

In adults, intensive blood glucose control with oral hypoglycemic agents and insulin has been demonstrated to substantially decrease the risk of microvascular complications (57). This study also found that treatment of hypertension in adults with type 2 diabetes significantly lowered the risk of cardiovascular disease (57).

Treatment of hyperlipidemia in patients with diabetes, as in nondiabetic patients, decreases the risk of macrovascular complications and should be part of the treatment regimen (58).

Management

The management of type 2 diabetes should be family based and include diabetes self-management, which encompasses the following (13):

1. Family involvement
2. Education, including a basic knowledge of pathophysiology and short- and long-term complications of diabetes
3. Nutrition and meal planning
4. Exercise
5. Pharmacologic management
6. Self-monitoring

Family Involvement

It cannot be overstated how important family involvement is in treating type 2 diabetes and obesity and their related comorbidities. In a study of children and adolescents with type 2 diabetes, direct supervision by adult family members had a positive effect on blood sugar control (59).

Education

It is vital for patients and families to understand the causes of type 2 diabetes and the impact of family history, obesity, and lifestyle on the course of the disease. Families should be encouraged to work together for lifestyle change. Education about nutrition, activity, and the effect of sedentary behavior can lay the groundwork for such change. Because most children and adolescents with type 2 diabetes will have family members with type 2 diabetes, it is important to understand how the family has approached this diagnosis. If older members of the family have developed a more passive approach to the disease, it is important to help the child and adolescent, along with their family, take a more proactive approach.

Nutrition

Even modest (10%) weight loss can improve glycemic control.

Generally, a balanced dietary approach with reduction of total calories, usually starting with the elimination of excess sugar, will begin to reverse the tendency toward weight gain and deterioration in glycemic control. The ADA position statement on nutritional recommendations in diabetes suggests use of the non-nutritive sweeteners approved by the Food and Drug Administration (FDA) (saccharin, aspartame, acesulfame potassium, sucralose) as long as they are consumed within the acceptable daily intake levels established by the FDA (60). If dyslipidemia is present, normalization of lipids is also a dietary goal. Less than 10% of the energy intake should be from saturated fats, and patients with low-density lipoprotein (LDL) cholesterol greater than or equal to 100 mg/dL may benefit from lowering saturated fat intake to less than 7% of energy intake. Dietary cholesterol intake should be less than 300 mg/day, and if LDL cholesterol is greater than 100 mg/dL, dietary cholesterol should be lowered to 200 mg/day (60). Protein intake should follow age-specific requirements. Although very large amounts of fiber may benefit insulin resistance, glycemic control, and plasma lipids, it is unclear if these benefits are achievable because of poor palatability and the gastrointestinal side effects of a large fiber load (60). Children and families should work with a nutritionist whenever possible to optimize and individualize dietary planning.

Weight loss decreases insulin resistance, reduces the tendency toward hyperglycemia and dyslipidemia, and lowers blood pressure. As in all cases of weight loss, a structured, intensive lifestyle program involving education, individualized counseling, reduced fat and energy intake, regular physical activity, and frequent patient contact is needed (60).

Physical Activity

Physical activity has been shown to correlate with lower fasting insulin and greater insulin sensitivity in children (61). In adults, low levels of physical activity have been associated with the future risk of type 2 diabetes (62). Because regular activity may not have been a part of the obese child's or adolescent's lifestyle before the diagnosis, scheduling a time for exercise or enrolling in a structured exercise program is beneficial. Clearly, reduction in television watching is important for both increasing activity and decreasing excess snacking (63,64).

Pharmacotherapy

The ADA suggests pharmacotherapy if the $HgbA_{1C}$ is greater than 7% (30). The first line of pharmacotherapy is metformin. Of the oral pharmacologic agents used in adults with type 2 diabetes, only metformin has been approved for use in children who are older than 10 years (53). Metformin decreases hepatic gluconeogenesis, increases insulin sensitivity, and lowers triglycerides and LDL cholesterol. Metformin raises insulin sensitivity in muscle by upregulating GLUT 4 activity and increasing insulin receptor tyrosine kinase activity. It has no effect on pancreatic insulin secretion but requires the presence of insulin to be effective (13). In a 5-year retrospective review of African American and Hispanic pubertal patients who presented with type 2 diabetes, 45% were able to keep their $HgbA_{1C}$ levels less than 7% with oral medications, which included metformin, 18% required insulin in addition to oral medications, and 37% did not require medication (65).

The most common side effect is gastrointestinal disturbance, including nausea, vomiting, a sense of fullness, constipation, and heartburn, which may diminish over time. The most serious side effect is lactic acidosis, occurring in patients with renal impairment or liver failure.

Patients with renal insufficiency, liver disease, alcohol abuse, hypoxemia and hypoperfusion, and sepsis should not use metformin. Metformin must be discontinued when the patient receives contrast dye and during serious illness (53). Temporary insulin therapy may be needed for severe symptoms at diagnosis, during acute intercurrent illness or steroid therapy, and perioperatively (53).

Vitamin B_{12} deficiency has been reported in adults in association with long-term use of metformin. Patients with this deficiency present with mild anemia, and some report having asthenia, peripheral neuropathy, and lower limb edema (66,67).

Additional oral agents used in adults are undergoing study in the pediatric age group. These agents include thiazolidinediones, sulfonylurea, meglitinides, acarbose, and α-glucosidase inhibitors.

Insulin therapy is often necessary to re-establish metabolic control. Combinations of long-acting and rapid-acting insulin are part of intensive insulin therapy in which both basal and bolus insulin are used to simulate normal insulin secretion. Insulin pump therapy may be used to accomplish this goal (53). Studies in adults show that beta cell function gradually deteriorates because of hyperglycemia, to the point at which oral agents can no longer induce insulin production, and that this occurs on average about 6 to 10 years after diagnosis. Therefore, supplementing oral agents with insulin, as soon as necessary to re-establish metabolic control, is recommended (53).

Monitoring

Ongoing monitoring should include measurements of the following:

- Glucose and $HgbA_{1C}$
- Blood urea nitrogen (BUN)/creatinine (Crt), liver function tests (if on metformin)
- Microalbuminuria
- Lipid levels
- Dilated eye examination
- Blood pressure
- Neurologic and foot examinations (49)

DIABETES-ASSOCIATED COMPLICATIONS

The degree and duration of hyperglycemia are associated with the risk for and development of diabetic microvascular and macrovascular complications. Certain populations of children have presented at diagnosis with evidence of increased cardiovascular risk (68). In adults, risk of the microvascular complications of retinopathy, nephropathy, and neuropathy can be decreased by intensive blood glucose control (57). Furthermore, the treatment of hypertension and hyperlipidemia lowered the risk of cardiovascular disease (57).

Cardiovascular Complications

The insulin resistance syndrome has been associated with risk factors for cardiovascular disease (69) and type 2 diabetes is considered a *major* risk factor for coronary artery disease. In obese children, dyslipidemia correlates with the degree of insulin resistance (70).

Elevated insulin levels increase renal sodium retention while increasing free water clearance and are linked with greater sympathetic nervous system activity and stimulation of avascular smooth muscle growth (71), increasing the risk for hypertension.

Lipid-Lowering Therapy

The ADA recommends that children and adolescents with type 2 diabetes should be screened for hyperlipidemia at diagnosis and early in the course of the disease after glycemic control is achieved. The most common cause of hyperlipidemia is continuing poor control of hyperglycemia. Optimal levels of lipids for children and adolescents with diabetes are as follows (72):

Total cholesterol <170 mg/dL
LDL cholesterol <100 mg/dL
HDL cholesterol >35 mg/dL
Triglycerides <150 mg/dL

Borderline levels are defined as
Total cholesterol 170–199 mg/dL
LDL cholesterol 110–129 mg/dL

Elevated levels are defined as
Total cholesterol >200 mg/dL
LDL cholesterol >130 mg/dL

It is now suggested that treatment for hyperlipidemia begin with the American Heart Association Step 2 diet. This diet holds dietary cholesterol below 200 mg/dL and saturated fat at less than 7% of total calories (72). Laboratory follow-up with fasting lipid profiles should be performed in the first 3 to 6 months after the initiation of treatment to monitor effectiveness of the dietary interventions and then yearly thereafter (72).

Pharmacotherapy has been recommended by the ADA in children older than 10 years to optimize the LDL cholesterol, if LDL levels stay greater than or equal to 160 mg/dL in children with obesity and a high risk of cardiovascular disease (diabetes, hypertension, and positive family history) (72).

Bile acid sequestrants can be used as treatment, but compliance may be low. The ADA (72) refers to two studies of statins (3-hydroxy-3-methylglutaryl coenzyme A reductase inhibitors) in adolescents. In the first study, sponsored by the drug company manufacturing the agent, simvastatin was used in postmenarchal girls and boys classified as Tanner II or greater with heterozygous familial hypercholesterolemia in a 48-week randomized controlled trial. None of these children had diabetes. The average BMI was 21 in boys and 22 in girls. LDL values were lowered by an average of 41%. Transient elevations of liver enzymes occurred in one case thought to be due to the drug and in one child with infectious mononucleosis. Elevated creatine phosphokinase (CPK) also was noted in a child taking erythromycin. Cholesterol is a precursor of the adrenal hormones cortisol and dihydroepiandrosterone (DHEAS) and the gonadal hormones testosterone and estradiol; in this study, significant reductions in DHEAS were found (73).

The second study was performed in boys with heterozygous familial hypercholesterolemia (74). LDL decreased 17% to 27%, depending on the dose, over 48 weeks. The authors note that

> Growth and sexual maturation assessed by Tanner staging and testicular volume were not significantly different between the lovastatin and placebo groups at 24 weeks ($P =$ .85) and 48 weeks ($P = .33$); neither were serum hormone levels or biochemical parameters of nutrition. However, the study was underpowered to detect significant differences in safety parameters. Serum vitamin E levels were reduced with lovastatin treatment consistent with reductions in LDL-C, the major carrier of vitamin E in the circulation.

The funding for this second study was not identified. The ADA recommends that when

> . . . statins are used, treatment should begin at the lowest available dose and dose increases should be based on LDL levels and side effects. Liver function tests (LFTs)

should be monitored and medication should be discontinued if LFTs are greater than three times the upper limit of normal. If there is any persistent complaint of significant muscle pain/muscle soreness, the medication should be discontinued to see if symptoms resolve. Routine monitoring of creatine phosphokinase levels is not felt to be helpful. In addition, the use of statins in sexually active adolescent females must be very carefully considered and the risks explicitly discussed, as these drugs are not approved in pregnancy (68).

If triglyceride levels are greater than 150 mg/dL, dietary therapy and glycemic control are the first line of treatment. Specific recommendations for triglyceride values greater than 1,000 mg/dL are to consider treating with a fibric acid medication. Smoking cessation, blood pressure control, and physical activity are also important in managing cardiac risk reduction (68).

Hypertension

Hypertension is a major risk factor for cardiovascular and renal disease. Treatment of hypertension is important and does not differ in children and adolescents with type 2 diabetes (see Chapter 7 for discussion of treatment) (68).

Polycystic Ovarian Syndrome

The prevalence of type 2 diabetes and IGT is increased in polycystic ovarian syndrome (PCOS) (75). Adolescent girls with PCOS have a 50% reduction in peripheral insulin sensitivity, abnormal first-phase insulin response, and lack of beta cell compensation with compensatory hyperinsulinemia (76).

Psychological Well-Being

Ensuring psychological well-being is a component of all therapeutic efforts involved in the treatment of type 2 diabetes. Depression has been associated with obesity in children and adolescents (77). In one study of a hospital-based urban pediatric population with type 2 diabetes, an increased frequency of neuropsychiatric disorders was found. Just over 19% of type 2 diabetes patients presenting for treatment had a diagnosed mental health disorder (78). More females than males were affected, but there was no ethnic, BMI, or demographic difference between affected and unaffected patients. Diagnoses included neurodevelopmental disorders, psychiatric illness, and behavioral disorders, with two thirds of patients prescribed psychotropic medications (78).

Additional Obesity-Related Comorbidities

It is worth noting that obese patients with type 2 diabetes are also at risk for other obesity-related comorbidities, such as sleep apnea and upper airway obstruction and NASH. In fact, a high prevalence of elevated liver function studies has been reported in a population of children with type 2 diabetes. Forty-eight percent had elevated serum transaminase levels, with 60% of these being more than twice the upper limit of normal. These elevations did not correlate with age, BMI, or HgbA$_{1C}$ (79).

ONGOING SUPPORT: CASE OF HJ

Initial Presentation

HJ is a 14-year-old African American young lady who is brought to your office by her mother because of the family's concern about diabetes. HJ's mother developed type 2 diabetes as a young adult and is now treated with insulin and has early diabetic retinopathy. HJ is not very happy about being at the doctor's, but you have some history with her because you have been struggling to help get her asthma under control.

You note that her weight is 152 lb (91st percentile) and height is 5 ft 1 in. (10th percentile). Her calculated BMI is 28.7, which places her above the 95th percentile and she has gained about 20 lb over the past year. You begin by asking about her eating and activity. She says little, so you discuss her daily routine with her. She is skipping breakfast and having lunch at school, which consists of a snack and soda. When HJ comes home from school, her mother notes, she is "starving" and eating "anything," which turns out to be leftovers or snack food. She drinks soda between meals. After school, she sometimes watches television and sometimes naps, working on her homework in between. The family sometimes cooks, sometimes orders take-out food, and the family members frequently eat separately. HJ says that she doesn't eat before bed, but her mother says she often finds dishes and snack wrappers in HJ's room. HJ had physical education last term in school, but she does not really spend time outside and has no extracurricular activities.

Catching up on the rest of the family history, you find that the maternal grandmother also has diabetes, as does the paternal grandfather. Numerous aunts and uncles have hypertension, and several great uncles have had coronary artery disease.

In the review of systems, you note she has asthma, which is poorly controlled, and an irregular menstrual cycle. On physical examination, you note her elevated BMI and a blood pressure of 128/86 mm Hg, which is greater than the 95th percentile for systolic and diastolic pressure. She has moderate acanthosis nigricans of her neck and axilla. Besides slight wheezing, she has no other positive physical findings.

You check HJ's blood glucose on the office glucometer and it is 105 mg/dL, and she has not eaten breakfast. You order a 2-hour glucose tolerance test with insulin; laboratory studies to evaluate her metabolic status with regard to her obesity [total cholesterol, HDL cholesterol, triglycerides, aspartate aminotransferase (AST), alanine aminotransferase (ALT), γ-glutamyltransferase (GGT)] and her possible PCOS (total testosterone, free testosterone, DHEAS, sex hormone binding globulin); and a metabolic panel.

You tell HJ and her mother about the risk for diabetes and PCOS as well as the blood pressure elevation. Her mother is upset and asks what they can do; HJ looks somewhat concerned and asks if she will need "shots."

You ask HJ what she knows about diabetes. She knows it concerns high "sugar." You explain insulin resistance and diabetes and inform HJ and her mother that with diet and activity change HJ can dramatically lower her risk for diabetes. You mention several things they might consider changing, such as eliminating or decreasing sugar-containing beverages, eating healthier after school snacks, and cooking at home. The mother says that HJ should stop drinking soda; you mention that it would be easier for HJ to stop if there were no sugar-containing beverages in the house. The mother says she thinks she can eliminate them, but HJ's father "won't like it." You ask HJ's mother to invite her father to come to the next visit.

You ask HJ if there is anything she can do to increase her activity; she says she does not know but mentions she likes to dance. You start with this and ask her to play a dance tape for 15 minutes/day and keep an activity log. You arrange to see HJ again in the clinic in 1 month.

About 1 week later, you receive a laboratory report for HJ. HJ's 2-hour glucose was 152 mg/dL, indicating IGT; her 2-hour insulin was 296 μU/mL, showing marked insulin resistance. As is typical of the lipid profile in insulin resistance, her cholesterol was mildly elevated at 186 mg/dL and her triglycerides were 215 mg/dL, with a low HDL cholesterol of 32 mg/dL. The results for liver function studies were normal. But her testosterone, free testosterone, and DHEAS were mildly elevated. Your nurse gives HJ's mother a call to report the results and to check on how the family is doing with eliminating soda and juice and increasing HJ's activity. The mother reports that all sugar-containing beverages are out of the house and HJ has been doing "some" dancing and has also gone out with her friends and walked the mall.

Second Visit

When HJ comes back for her visit, her weight has decreased by 1.5 lb and her blood pressure is 122/79 mm Hg (systolic between the 90% and 95% and diastolic <90%). Her fasting glucose is 99 mg/dL. HJ and her mother report that HJ has not had any soda or juice, and the mother has removed sugared drinks from the house. HJ's father has been supportive (he is drinking his regular soda at his work). HJ has done some dancing and gone out with friends a little more, and you discuss other possible activity options, such as a dance class, after school activity, and/or a volunteer job. You give them diet and activity records to monitor, asking them to fax the records weekly, and arrange to see HJ again in 1 month. You also notice that HJ is more communicative, and she and her mother are less irritable with each other; you comment on this and congratulate them on making these lifestyle changes.

Follow-up Visits

You tell HJ and her mother that you plan to see HJ monthly until her laboratory studies and menstrual cycle normalize and they feel they have made changes they can sustain.

REFERENCES

1. Srinivasan SR, Myers L, Berenson GS. Predictability of childhood adiposity and insulin for developing insulin resistance syndrome (syndrome X) in young adulthood: the Bogalusa Heart Study. *Diabetes.* 2002;51(1):204–209.
2. Hassink S. Problems in childhood obesity. *Prim Care.* 2003;31(2):357–374.
3. Reaven GM. 1988 Banting lecture. Role of insulin resistance in human disease. *Diabetes.* 1988;37:1595–1607.
4. Daskalopoulou SS, Athyros VG, Kolovou GD, Anagnostopoulou KK, Mikhailidis DP. Definitions of metabolic syndrome: where are we now? *Curr Vasc Pharmacol.* 2006;4(3):185–197.
5. Santoro N, Cirillo G, Amato A, Luongo C, Raimondo P, D'aniello A, Perrone L, Mairaglia Del Giudice E. Insulin gene VNTR genotype and metabolic syndrome in childhood. *Obes J Clin Endocrinol Metab.* 2006;Jul 25.
6. Boney CM, Verma A, Tucker R, Vohr BR. Metabolic syndrome in childhood: association with birth weight, maternal obesity, and gestational diabetes mellitus. *Pediatrics.* 2005;115(3):e290–e296.
7. Sinha R, Fisch G, Teague B, Tamborlane WV, Banyas B, Allen K, Savoye M, Rieger V, Taksali S, Barbetta G, Sherwin RS, Caprio S. Prevalence of impaired glucose tolerance among children and adolescents with marked obesity. *N Engl J Med.* 2002;346:802–810.
8. Ten S, Maclaren N. Insulin resistance syndrome in children. *J Clin Endocrinol Metab.* 2004;89: 2526–2539.
9. American Diabetes Association. Type 2 diabetes in children and adolescents. *Diabetes Care.* 2000; 23(3):381–389.
10. Rosenbloom AL, Joe JR, Young RS, Winter WE. Emerging epidemic of type 2 diabetes in youth. *Diabetes Care.* 1999;22(2):345–354.
11. Libman I, Arslanian S. Type 2 diabetes in childhood: the American perspective. *Horm Res.* 2003; 59(Suppl 1):69–76.
12. Neal JV. Diabetes mellitus: a thrifty genotype rendered detrimental by "progress." *Am J Hum Genet.* 1962;14:353–362.
13. Pinhas-Hamiel O, Zeitler P. Advances in epidemiology and treatment of type 2 diabetes in children. *Adv Pediatr.* 2005;52:223–259.
14. Arslanian S. Type 2 diabetes in children: clinical aspects and risk factors. *Horm Res.* 2002;(Suppl 1):19–28.
15. Alberti G, Zimmet P, Shaw J, Bloomgarden Z, Kaufman F, Silink M; for the Consensus Workshop Group. Type 2 diabetes in the young:the evolving epidemic. The International Diabetes Federation Consensus Workshop.*Diabetes Care.* 2004;27(7):1798–1811.
16. Kaufman FR. Type 2 diabetes in children and youth. *Endocrinol Metab Clin North Am.* 2005;34(3): 659–676.
17. Watson RT, Pessin JE. Intracellular organization of insulin signaling and GLUT4 translocation. *Recent Prog Horm Res.* 2001;56:175–194 .
18. Weiss R, Dufour S, Taksali SE, Tamborlane WV, Petersen KF, Bonadonna RC, Boselli L, Barbetta G, Allen K, Rife F, Savoye M, Dziura J, Sherwin R, Shulman GL, Caprio S. Prediabetes in obese youth: a syndrome of impaired glucose tolerance, severe insulin resistance, and altered myocellular and abdominal fat partitioning. *Lancet.* 2003;362:951–957.
19. Porte D Jr. Banting Lecture 1990: Beta cells in type II diabetes mellitus. *Diabetes.* 1991;40(2): 166–180.
20. Barroso I. Genetics of type 2 diabetes. *Diabet Med.* 2005;22(5):517–535.
21. Goran ML, Ball CGC, Cruz ML.Obesity and risk of type 2 diabetes and cardiovascular disease in children and adolescents. *J Clin Endocrinol Metab.* 2002;88(1):192–195.
22. Caprio S, Hyman LD, Limb C, McCarthy S, Lange R, Sherwin RS, Shulman G, Tamborlane WV. Central adiposity and its metabolic correlates in obese adolescent girls. *Am J Physiol.* 1995; 269(1Pt1):E118–E126.
23. Moreno LA, Pineda I, Rodriquez G, Fleta J, Sarria A, Bueno M, et al. Waist circumference for the screening of the metabolic syndrome in children. *Acta Pediatr.* 2002;91:1307–1312.
24. Cruz ML, Bergman RN, Goran MI. Unique effect of visceral fat on insulin sensitivity in obese Hispanic children with a family history of type 2 diabetes. *Diabetes Care.* 2002;25(9):1631–1636.
25. Krssak M, Falk Perersen K, Dresner A, DiPietro L, Vogel SM, Rothman DL, Roden M, Shulman GI. Intramyocellular lipid concentrations are correlated with insulin sensitivity in humans; 1H-NMR spectroscopy study. *Diabetologia.* 1999;42(1):113–116.

26. Moran O, Phillip M. Leptin: obesity, diabetes and other peripheral effects—a review. *Pediatr Diabetes.* 2003;4(2):101–109.
27. Arslenian S, Suprasongsin C. Differences in the in vivo insulin secretion and sensitivity in healthy black vs. white adolescents. *J Pediatr.* 1996;129(3):440–444.
28. Svec F, Nastasi K, Hilton C, Bao W, Srinivasan SR, Berenson GS. Black-white contrasts in insulin levels during pubertal development: the Bogalusa Heart Study. *Diabetes.* 1992;41(3):313–317.
29. Perusse L, Rankinen T, Zuberi A, Chagnon YC, Weisnagel SF, Argyropoulos G, Walts B, Snyder EE, Bouchard C. The human obesity gene map: the 2004 update. *Obes Res.* 2005;13:381–490.
30. American Diabetes Association. Type 2 diabetes in children and adolescents. *Pediatrics.* 2000; 105(3Pt1):671–680.
31. Libman I, Arslanian SA. Type 2 diabetes mellitus: no longer just adults. *Pedatr Ann.* 1999;28(9): 589–593.
32. McIntyre EA, Walker M. Genetics of type 2 diabetes and insulin resistance: knowledge from human studies. *Clin Endocrinol(Oxf).* 2002;57(3):303–311.
33. Zimmet PZ. Kelly West Lecture 1991. Challenges in diabetes epidemiology from west to the rest. *Diabetes Care.* 1992;15(2):232–352.
34. Buinauskiene J, Baliutaviciene D, Zalinkevicius R. Glucose tolerance of 2 to 5 year old offspring of diabetic mothers. *Pediatr Diabetes.* 2004;5(3):143–146.
35. Hales CN, Barker DJ. Type 2 (non insulin dependent) diabetes mellitus; the thrifty phenotype hypothesis. *Diabetologia.* 1992;35(7):595–601.
36. Weiss PAM, Scholz HS, Haas J, Tamussino KF, Seissler J, Borkenstein MH. Long term follow up of infants of mothers with type I diabetes: evidence for hereditary and non hereditary transmission of diabetes and precursors. *Diabetes Care.* 2000;23(7):905–911.
37. Plagemann A, Harder T, Franke K, Kohlhoff R. Long-term impact of neonatal breast feeding on body weight and glucose tolerance in children of diabetic mothers. *Diabetes Care.* 2002;25(1):16–22.
38. Forsen T, Eriksson J, Tuomilehto J, Reunanen A, Osmond C, Barker D. The fetal and childhood growth of persons who develop type 2 diabetes. *Ann Intern Med.* 2000;133(3):176–182.
39. Yajnik C. Interactions of perturbations in intrauterine growth and growth during childhood and risk of adult onset disease. *Proc Nutr Soc.* 2000;59(2):257–265.
40. Ong KK, Dunger DB. Birth weight, infant growth and insulin resistance. *Eur J Endocrinol.* 2004; 151(3):U131–U139.
41. Eriksson JG, Forsen T, Tuomileto J, Osmond C, Barker DJP. Early adiposity rebound in children and risk of type 2 diabetes in adult life. *Diabetologia.* 2003;46(2):190–194.
42. Hales CN, Barker DJ. The thrifty phenotype hypothesis. *Br Med Bull.* 2001;60:5–20.
43. Arslanian S. Type 2 diabetes mellitus in children. Pathophysiology and risk factors. *J Pediatr Endocrinol Metab.* 2000;13 (Suppl 6):1385–1394.
44. Caprio S, Plewe G, Diamond MP, Simonson DC, Boulware SD, Sherwin RS, Tamborlane WV. Increased insulin secretion in puberty: a compensatory response to reductions in insulin sensitivity. *J Pediatr.* 1989;114(6):963–967.
45. The Expert Committee on the Diagnosis and Classification of Diabetes Mellitus. Report of the Expert Committee on the Diagnosis and Classification of Diabetes Mellitus. *Diabetes Care.* 2003;Suppl 1:S5–S20.
46. Genuth S, Alberti KG, Bennett P, Defronzo R, Kahn R, Kitzmiller J, Knowler WC, Lebovitz H, Lernmark A, Nathan D, Palmer J, Rizza R, Saudek C, Shaw J, Steffes M, Stern M, Tuomilehto J, Zimmet P. Expert Committee on the Diagnosis and Classification of Diabetes Mellitus. Follow-up report on the diagnosis of diabetes mellitus. *Diabetes Care.* 2003;26:3160–3167.
47. Gomez-Diaz R, Aguilar-Salinas CA, Moran Villota S, Barradas-Gonzalez R, Herrera-Marquez R, Lopez MC, Kkumate J, Wacher NH. Lack of agreement between the revised criteria of impaired fasting glucose and impaired glucose tolerance in children with excess body weight. *Diabetes Care.* 2004;27:2229–2233.
48. Tuomilehto J, Lindstrom J, Eriksson JG, Valle TT, Hamalainen H, Iiane-Parrika P, Keinanen-Kiukaanniemi S, Laakso M, Louheranta A, Rastas M, Salminen V, Uustiupa M. Finnish Diabetes Prevention Study Group. Prevention of type 2 diabetes mellitus by changes in lifestyle among subjects with impaired glucose tolerance. *N Engl J Med.* 2001;344(18):343–350.
49. Ayer T, Levitsky LL. Type 2 diabetes: an epidemic disease in childhood. *Curr Opin Pediatr.* 2003;15(4):411–415.
50. Gungor N, Arslanian S. Pathophysiology of type 2 diabetes in children and adolescents: treatment implications *Treat Endocrinol.* 2002;1:359–371.

51. Stuart CA, Pate CJ, Peters EJ. Prevalence of acanthosis nigricans in an unselected population. *Am J Med.* 1989;87:269–272.
52. Williams CL, Hayman LL, Daniels SR, Robinson TN Steinberer J, Paridon S, Bazzare T. Cardiovascular health in childhood. A statement for health professionals from the Committee on Atherosclerosis, Hypertension and Obesity in the Young of the Council on Cardiovascular Disease in the Young AHA. *Circulation.* 2002;106(1):143–160.
53. Miller JL, Silverstein JH. The management of type 2 diabetes mellitus in children and adolescents. *J Pediatr Endocrinol Metab.* 2005;18(2):111–123.
54. Pinhas-Hamiel O, Dolan LM, Danials SR, Standiford D, Khoury PR, Zeitler P. Increased incidence of non-insulin dependent diabetes mellitus among adolescents. *J Pediatr.* 1996;128(5pt1):608–615.
55. Morales AE, Rosenbloom AL. Death caused by hyperglycemic hyperosmolar state at the onset of type 2 diabetes. *J Pediatr.* 2004;144(2):270–273.
56. Rubin HM, Kramer R, Drash A. Hyperosmolality complicating diabetes mellitus in childhood. *J Pediatr.* 1969;74(4):177–186.
57. UK Prospective Diabetes Study (UKPDS) Group. Intensive blood-glucose control with sulphonylureas or insulin compared with conventional treatment and risk of complications in patients with type 2 diabetes (UKPDS33). *Lancet.* 1998;3352(9131):837–853.
58. Laakso M. Lipids in type 2 diabetes. *Semin Vasc Med.* 2002;2:59–66.
59. Bradshaw B. The role of the family in managing therapy in minority children with diabetes mellitus. *J Pediatr Endocrinol Metab.* 2002;15(Suppl 1):547–551.
60. American Diabetes Association Task Force for Writing Nutrition Principles and Recommendations for the Management of Diabetes and Related Complications. American Diabetes Association Position Statement: Evidence based nutrition principles and recommendations for the treatment and prevention of diabetes and related complications. *J Am Diet Assoc.* 2002;102:109–118.
61. Schmitz KH, Jacobs DR, Hong CP, et al. Association of physical activity with insulin sensitivity in children. *Int J Obes.* 2002;26:1310–1316.
62. Helmrich SP, Ragland DR, Leung RW, Paffenbarger RS. Physical activity and reduced occurrence of non insulin dependent diabetes mellitus. *N Engl J Med.* 1991;325(3):147–152.
63. Epstein LH, Valoski AM, Vara LS, McCurley J, Wisniewski L, Kalarchian MA, Klein KR, Shrager LR. Effects of decreasing sedentary behavior and increasing activity on weight change in obese children. *Health Psychol.* 1995;14(2):109–115.
64. Robinson TN. Television viewing and childhood obesity. *Pediatr Clin North Am.* 2001;48(4):1017–1025.
65. Grinstein G, Muzumdar R, Aponte L, Vuquin P, Saenger P, Di Martino-Nardi J. Presentation and 5 year follow up of type 2 diabetes mellitus in African American and Caribbean-Hispanic adolescents. *Horm Res.* 2003;60:121–126.
66. Andres E, Noel E, Goichot B. Metformin-associated vitamin B_{12} deficiency. *Arch Intern Med.* 2002;162(19):2251–2252.
67. Stowers JM, Smith OA. Vitamin B_{12} and metformin. *Br Med J.* 1971;3:246–247.
68. Fagot-Campagna A, Knowler WC, Pettitt DJ, Engelgau MM, Burrows NR, Geiss LS, Valdez R, Beckles GL, Saadine J, Gregg EW, Williamson DF, Narayan DM. Type 2 diabetes among North American children and adolescents: an epidemiologic review and a public health perspective. *Pediatrics.* 2000;136(5):644–672.
69. Steinberger J. Insulin resistance and cardiovascular risk in the pediatric patient. *Prog Pediatr Cardiol.* 2001;12(12):169–175.
70. Steinberger J, Moorehead C, Kntch V, Roccini AP. Relationship between insulin resistance and abnormal lipid profile in obese adolescents. *J Pediatr.* 1995;126(5Pt1):690–695.
71. Steinberger J. Diagnosis of the metabolic syndrome in children. *Curr Opin Lipidol.* 2003;14(6):555–559.
72. American Diabetes Association. Management of dyslipidemia in children and adolescents with diabetes. *Diabetes Care.* 2003;26(7):2194–2197.
73. De Jongh S, Ose L, Szamosi T, Gagne C, Lambert M, Scott R, Perron P, Dobbelaere D, Saborio M, Tuohy MB, Stepanavage M, Sapre A, Gumbiner B, Mercuri M, van Trotsenburg AS, Bakker HD, Kastelein JJ; Simvastatin in Children Study Group. Efficacy and safety of statin therapy in children with familial hypercholesterolemia: a randomized, double-blind, placebo-controlled trial with simvastatin. *Circulation.* 2002;106(17):2231–2237.
74. Stein EA, Illingworth DR, Kwiterovich PO Jr, Liacouras CA, Siimes MA, Jacobson MS, Brewster TG, Hopkins P, Davidson M, Graham K, Arensman F, Knopp RH, DuJovne C, Williams CL, Isaac-

sohn JL, Jacobsen CA, Laskarzewski PM, Ames S, Gormley GJ. Efficacy and safety of lovastatin in adolescent males with heterozygous familial hypercholesterolemia: a randomized controlled trial. *JAMA.* 1999;281(2):137–144.

75. Lewy VD, Donadian K, Witchel SF, Arslanian S. Early metabolic abnormalities in adolescent girls with PCOS. *J Pediatr.* 2001;138:38–41.

76. Arslanian SA, Levy VD, Danadian K. Glucose intolerance in obese adolescents with polycystic ovary syndrome: roles in insulin resistance and B cell dysfunction and risk of cardiovascular disease. *J Clin Endocrinol Metab.* 2001;86:66–71.

77. Goodman E, Whitaker RC. A prospective study of the role of depression in the development and persistence of adolescent obesity. *Pediatrics.* 2002;110(3):497–504.

78. Levitt Katz LE, Swami S, Abraham M, Murphy KM, Jawad AF, McKnight-Menci H, Berkowitz R. Neuropsychiatric disorders at the presentation of type 2 diabetes mellitus in children. *Pediatr Diabetes.* 2005;6(2):84–89.

79. Nadeau KJ, Klingensmith G, Zeitler P. Type 2 diabetes in children is frequently associated with elevated alanine aminotransferase. *J Pediatr Gastroenterol Nutr.* 2005;41(1):94–98.

9

Orthopedic Complications

Slipped capital femoral epiphysis (SCFE) and Blount's disease (tibia vara) are becoming more prevalent as the rates of obesity and morbid obesity increase.

Skeletal maturation is a feature of adolescent development, with closure of the growth plate signaling the attainment of adult height. Obese children are susceptible to unique orthopedic problems, which occur during growth.

SCFE is the most common hip disorder of adolescence. Prevalence rates as high as 10.08 per 100,000 have been reported in the 1970s in the northeast United States (1). In data from the National Inpatient Sample from 1993 to 2000 (data collected from 1,000 hospitals to approximate a 20% sample of U.S. hospital discharges), 4,924 patients were treated for SCFE from ages 7 to 17 years (2). It has also been observed that 70% of children having SCFE had weights above the 80th percentile for age (3). In children from 8 to 18 years of age who had radiologic studies to rule out SCFE, a retrospective review of charts from 1994 to 2004 found that more children were obese or at risk for obesity (95.3%) who were diagnosed with SCFE than children with symptoms due to other causes (41.3%) (4).

The incidence of SCFE is highest during puberty, with the peak in incidence in boys from 12 to 15 years and in girls 10 to 13 years (5). In an international study of SCFE, relative risk of disease (compared with the Caucasian population) was highest in the Polynesian population, relative risk (RR) 4.5, followed by 2.2 for black, 1.05 for American Indian, 0.5 for Indonesian-Malay, and 0.1 for Indo-Mediterranean children (6). Long-term consequences of SCFE can include the following (4):

- Degenerative hip disease
- Gait abnormalities
- Chondrolysis
- Avascular osteonecrosis

Idiopathic SCFE is associated with obesity.
Atypical SCFE can be caused by the following:

- Hypothyroidism
- Hypogonadism
- Renal osteodystrophy

104

- Osteomalacia
- Radiation therapy
- Chemotherapy

Adolescent tibia vara, or Blount's disease, is also more common in obese than in normal weight adolescents; up to two thirds of patients with Blount's disease are obese (7).

SLIPPED CAPITAL FEMORAL EPIPHYSIS

Definitions

- **Slipped capital femoral epiphysis**—Posterior and inferior slip of the proximal femoral epiphysis on the metaphysis (femoral neck) occurring through the zone of hypertrophic cartilage (physeal plate) (8).
- **Chondrolysis**—A process of progressive cartilage degeneration resulting in joint space narrowing and loss of motion, most frequently observed as a complication of SCFE (9).

Etiology

The pathology of SCFE involves a slip through the hypertrophic zone of the femoral growth plate. The growth plate includes undifferentiated or reserve cartilage cells, proliferating cartilage cells, and hypertrophic or maturing cartilage cells. In the undifferentiated zone, cartilage cells are in a resting state immediately adjacent to the epiphysis. Germinal cells from this layer supply the developing cartilage cells to increase the width of the growth plate.

The proliferative zone is where chondrocytes are actively growing and being aligned in columns to increase bone length. The hypertrophic or maturational zone is where chondrocytes terminally differentiate and mineralization begins. This is the weakest part of the growth plate (10,11) (Fig. 9.1).

The preferential site of slipping within the epiphysis is a zone of hypertrophic cartilage cells under the influence of both gonadal hormones and growth hormone (12). The exact cause of SCFE is unknown. SCFE often occurs at peak height velocity during puberty (13). The most common form of SCFE is seen in obese adolescents, who in some series have been slightly taller than their peers and have undergone slower than average skeletal maturation (5). Additional studies have shown that the age of onset of SCFE is younger with greater degrees of obesity (6).

Growth hormone stimulates the production of insulin-like growth factors (IGFs), which stimulate chondrocyte proliferation in the growth plate (13). Growth hormone has been found to stimulate local synthesis of IGFs by chondrocytes in rats (14). Futami (15) described features on magnetic resonance imaging (MRI) of a "preslip" that involved physeal widening. Lalaji et al. (16) described similar changes in two patients presenting with hip pain prior to the progression to a slip. Pathologically, chondrocyte degeneration and death have been noted throughout the hypertrophic

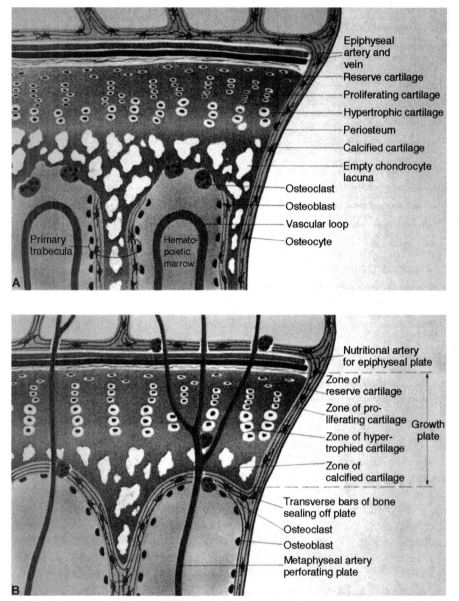

FIG. 9.1. Anatomy of the growth (epiphyseal) plate. **A:** Normal growing epiphyseal plate. The epiphysis is separated from the epiphyseal plate by transverse plates of bone that seal the plate so that it grows only toward the metaphysis. The various zones of cartilage are illustrated. As the calcified cartilage migrates toward the metaphysis, the chondrocytes die, and the lacunae are empty. At the interface of the epiphyseal plate and the metaphysis, osteoclasts bore into the calcified cartilage, accompanied by a capillary loop from the metaphyseal vessels. Osteoblasts follow the osteoclasts and lay down osteoid on the cartilage core, thereby forming the primary spongiosum, or primary trabeculae. **B:** Normal closure. The epiphyseal cartilage has ceased to grow, and metaphyseal vessels penetrate the cartilage plate. Transverse bars of bone separate the plate from the metaphysis. (From Rubin E, Farber JL. *Pathology Image Collection.* Philadelphia: Lippincott Williams & Wilkins;2000:Figure 26.9.)

and proliferative zones of SCFE growth plates (10,11). Adamczyck et al. (17) found a high incidence of apoptosis in SCFE growth plates from chronic slips when compared with normal growth plates. The reason for this is unknown, but they hypothesized that apoptosis occurred prior to the slip, weakening the growth plate and making it more susceptible to increased stress. In a review of patients with SCFE, 25% of those tested had low triiodothyronine levels, 76% of those tested had low testosterone levels, and 87% in this group also had low growth hormone levels, possibly reflecting subtle hormonal influences in this population (3).

Additional risk factors for SCFE include the following:

- Renal failure
- History of radiation therapy
- Primary hypothyroidism (18)
- Use of gonadotropin-releasing hormone agonists
- Growth hormone deficiency (treated or untreated) (9,19,20)

One study also found that levels of midportion parathyroid hormone (M-PTH) and 1,25-dihydroxy vitamin D (1,25-(OH) 2D), which are involved in growth-plate chondrogenesis and matrix mineralization, were significantly lower in patients with SCFE than in controls. In patients with initially low levels of M-PTH and 1,25-(OH) 2D, all levels returned to normal within a year after the onset of disease (21).

Most risk factors have been found to play a role in either decreasing the strength of the epiphyseal plate or increasing the amount of shearing stress to which the plate is subjected at the time it is most vulnerable (5). There have been cases of familial SCFE; Rennie (22) observed 12 adolescents with SCFE who also had an affected family member.

Clinical Manifestations

Obesity is clearly a predisposing factor in SCFE. In a study of 106 children presenting with SCFE, those affected had a mean body mass index (BMI) of 29.2, at an average age of 11.7 years. Ninety-five percent of children were greater than the 85th percentile for BMI and 81% were greater than the 95th percentile for BMI for age and gender (23). Obesity has been associated with a younger age at diagnosis. In a study from Michigan, 67% of patients diagnosed with SCFE were obese. The obese children were significantly younger at the time of the diagnosis of the slip (12 ± 1.6 years) than were the nonobese children (13 ± 1.6 years) (24). Bilateral slips may also be more common in obese children. In the same study, half the children had bilateral involvement on diagnosis, and half had only one hip affected. The children who went on to have a slip of the contralateral hip were more likely to be obese. The average time between diagnosis of the first and second slip was 1 ± 0.9 years (range 1–5 years). The diagnosis of the contralateral slip was made in 88% of the children within 18 months of the first slips (24).

In a study of bone maturation in children with SCFE, more than 82% of whom were greater than 1 SD above average weight and 54% greater than 3 SD above average weight, bone ages were found to be advanced in younger children and delayed in older children. In this study the average chronologic age was 13.6 ± 1.7 years for boys and 12.0 ± 1.4 years for girls, with 42% having a bone age corresponding to chronologic age (± 6 months). In 28%, bone age was advanced more than 6 months, and 30% had delay in mean bone age of more than 6 months (25). There is also a suggestion that chronic weight gain can increase the likelihood of a slip. In a study of BMI and SCFE, BMI values were increased starting from age 2 through age 14 in children with SCFE (26).

Increased repetitive stress and stress from injury have also been proposed as etiologic factors for SCFE. In a study from Japan, a history of injury was reported for 31.8% of children with SCFE. Seasonal variations in numbers of patients have been noted in relation to sports participation (27).

Endocrine disorders, particularly hypothyroidism and growth hormone deficiency, may alter age of onset of SCFE. In children with endocrine disorders, the average age at diagnosis of SCFE was 15.3 ± 5.3 years. This group of children was also noted to have discrepant bone/chronologic age, 11.6 ± 3.0 versus 16.5 ± 6.5 years, with a wider range of age at presentation (7–35 years) and a greater rate of bilateral involvement (61%) (28).

Slips can be either stable or unstable. A slip is considered stable if walking and weight bearing are still possible and unstable if walking is impossible regardless of the duration of symptoms (29). An unstable slip may present acutely, sometimes after a sports injury or fall, and it behaves more like a fracture. Unstable SCFE cases make up about 10% to 15% of the total cases of SCFE. Management of unstable SCFE is associated with most of the complications, including avascular necrosis and chondrolysis (29).

Evaluation

Early signs and symptoms of SCFE may be mild, with only vague complaints of pain and slight loss of internal rotation.

It is extremely important to ask about knee, groin, thigh, or hip pain in the history because children with early slips may not be reported.

As the slip progresses, loss of internal rotation, flexion, and abduction becomes even more apparent on examination and the gait becomes more painful. Obligate external rotation of the lower extremity is observed when the involved hip is flexed and can occur early in the course when radiologic changes are minimal (30). A child with a stable SCFE may give a history of intermittent pain and limping over weeks or even months. Pain may be localized to the thigh, groin, or knee because of the passage of sensory cutaneous nerves close to the hip capsule (31).

Delay in diagnosis has been correlated with the occurrence of knee and/or distal thigh pain, Medicaid coverage, and stable slips (31). In the same study, the median delay in diagnosis was 8 weeks, with a range of 0 to 111 weeks. There was a significant relationship between a longer delay in diagnosis and greater slip severity. There were no significant associations between diagnostic delay and age, gender, side of slip, or weight (31).

If a slip is suspected, no passive motion should be attempted, to avoid displacing the epiphysis (32). The child should be made non–weight-bearing right away and referred to an orthopedic surgeon for immediate correction. Diagnosis is made using an anteroposterior radiograph of the pelvis which includes both hips (Fig. 9.2). Findings of a widened growth plate and posterior slipping of the epiphysis are diagnostic. A line drawn along the anterior femoral neck should intersect the epiphysis in a normal hip (33). In a recent study, a lateral radiograph was also used to further define a subtle slip or examine the contralateral hip and was found to be more sensitive than the anteroposterior view in detecting an abnormality of the slipping angle (34).

MRI can be used to diagnose SCFE and to detect a widened growth plate and edema in preslip conditions (35). Clinical suspicion is paramount in making the diagnosis of SCFE, with radiologic studies used as confirmatory tests.

Treatment

The first aim of treatment is to prevent further slipping of the epiphysis. Suspicion of a slip is an orthopedic emergency, so consultation should be immediate. Pinning of the hip or hips results in good functional improvement. The risk of degenerative arthritis increases with the severity of the slip, making early diagnosis and treatment crucial. Avascular necrosis is the most serious complication, hastening the deterioration of the hip and requiring hip reconstruction or replacement (36).

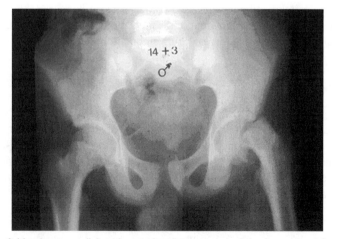

FIG. 9.2. Left hip shows medial and posterior displacement of the femoral epiphysis through the growth plate relative to the femoral neck. (Courtesy of Dr. Richard Bowen, Wilmington, Delaware.)

Complications

Chondrolysis is a process of progressive cartilage degeneration resulting in joint space narrowing and loss of motion, most frequently observed as a complication of SCFE (37). Higher immunoglobulin and C3 complement levels have been noted in SCFE patients who developed chondrolysis (38). A correlation has been found between "persistent" pin penetration of the femoral head after SCFE pinning and chondrolysis (39).

Avascular necrosis is an uncommon but serious complication of SCFE and may result in osteoarthritis (39a).

BLOUNT'S DISEASE (TIBIA VARA)

Definition

- **Blount's disease**—Medial bowing of the tibia (tibia vara) resulting from overgrowth of the proximal tibial metaphysis.

Etiology

There are four types of tibia vara: (a) infantile tibia vara occurs between the ages of 1 and 4 years, (b) juvenile tibia vara is caused by partial closure of the growth plate due to trauma or infection between the ages of 6 and 13, (c) adolescent-onset tibia vara due to obesity, and (d) tibia vara from other causes (40) (personal communication, R. Bowen, Orthopedics Department, A.I. duPont Hospital for Children, Wilmington, Delaware, May 2006). The exact mechanism of adolescent tibia vara due to obesity is not known. In a study of gait abnormalities in obese children, it was found that the gait deviation developed to compensate for increased thigh circumference could result in increased loading of the medial compartment of the knee, generating pathologic compressive forces during ambulation (41).

Clinical Manifestations

Patients present with medial bowing of the tibia. Clinical presentation can include pain and tenderness over the medial prominence of the proximal tibia, abnormal gait, and leg length discrepancy with shortening of the affected leg. X-ray studies confirm the findings (Fig. 9.3). Histologically, the usual columnar organization of the cartilage cells is disrupted with areas of acellular fibrous cartilage and abnormal groups of capillary vessels.

Treatment

Surgical osteotomy corrects the deformity.

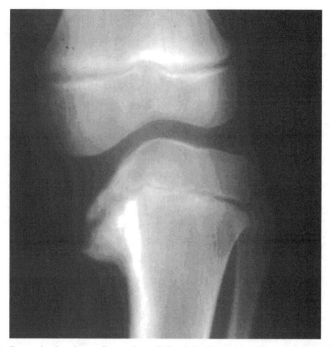

FIG. 9.3. Radiograph showing collapsed medial epiphysis and beaking of tibia in Blount's disease. (Courtesy of Dr. Richard Bowen, Wilmington, Delaware.)

IMPACT ON WEIGHT MANAGEMENT

Even common orthopedic injuries can become more complex for obese children and adolescents. They have been found to have a greater rate of persistent symptoms after ankle sprain than normal weight children. Symptoms include persistent pain, swelling, or weakness at 6 weeks and 6 months postinjury.

For every unit increase of BMI, the risk of having long-term morbidity increases 0.66% (42).

Gait abnormalities can be present following SCFE and further impair a patient's ability to participate in exercise. More severe slips have a higher correlation with abnormal gait. However, children with slip angles less than 30 degrees do not have any significant difference in gait than age- and weight-matched controls (43), further emphasizing the importance of early diagnosis and treatment.

REFERENCES

1. Kelsey JL, Keggi KJ, Southwick WO. The incidence and distribution of slipped capital femoral epiphysis in Connecticut and Southwestern United States. *J Bone Joint Surg Am.* 1970;52:1203–1216.
2. Brown D. Seasonal variation of slipped capital femoral epiphysis in the United States. *J Pediatr Orthop.* 2004;24:139–143.

3. Wilcox PC, Weiner DS, Leigh B. Maturation factors in slipped capital femoral epiphysis. *J Pediatr Orthop.* 1988;8:196–200.
4. Manoff EM, Banffy MB, Winell JJ. Relationship between body mass index and slipped capital femoral epiphysis. *J Pediatr Orthop.* 2005;25:744–746.
5. Kelsey JL. Epidemiology of slipped capital femoral epiphysis: a review of the literature. *Pediatrics.* 1973;51:1042–1050.
6. Loder R. The demographics of slipped capital femoral epiphysis: an international multicenter study. *Clin Orthop Rel Res.* 1996;322:8–17.
7. Dietz WH. Health consequences of obesity in youth: childhood predictors of adult disease. *Pediatrics.* 1998;101(3 Pt 2):518–525.
8. Busch MT, Morrissy RT. Slipped capital femoral epiphysis. *Orthop Clin North Am.* 1987;18(4): 637–647.
9. Yarbrough R, Gross R. Chondrolysis: an update. *J Pediatr Orthop.* 2005;25:702–704.
10. Agamanolis DP, Weiner DS, Lloyd JK. Slipped capital femoral epiphysis: a pathological study I. A light microscopic and histochemical study of 21 cases. *J Pediatr Orthop.* 1985;5:40–46.
11. Agamanolis DP, Weiner DS, Lloyd JK. Slipped capital femoral epiphysis: a pathological study II. An ultra structural study of 23 cases. *J Pediatr Orthop.* 1985;5:47–58.
12. Kempers MJ, Noordam C, Rouwe CW, Otten BJ. Can GRRH –agonist treatment cause slipped capital femoral epiphysis? *J Pediatr Endocrinol Metab.* 2001;14:729–734.
13. Jingushi S, Suenaga E. Slipped capital femoral epiphysis: etiology and treatment. *J Orthop Sci.* 2004;9:214–219.
14. Izumi T, Shida J, Jingushi S, Hotokebuchi T, Sugioka Y. Administration of growth hormone modulates the gene expression of basic fibroblast growth factor in rat costal cartilage, both in vivo and in vitro. *Mol Cell Endocrinol.* 1995;112(1):95–99.
15. Futami T, Suzuki S, Seto Y, Kashiwagi N. Sequential magnetic resonance imaging in slipped capital femoral epiphysis: assessment of preslip in the contralateral hip. *J Pediatr Orthop B.* 2001;1094:298–303.
16. Lalaji A, Umans H, Schneider R, Mintz D, Leilbling MS, Haramati N. MRI features of confirmed "pre slip" capital femoral epiphysis: a report of two cases. *Skeletal Radiol.* 2002;31(6):362–365.
17. Adamczyck MJ, Weiner DS, Nugent A, McBurney D, Horton W. Increased chondrocyte apoptosis in growth plates from children with slipped capital femoral epiphysis. *J Pediatr Orthop.* 2005;25: 440–444.
18. Loder RT, Greenfield ML. Clinical characteristics of children with atypical and idiopathic slipped capital femoral epiphysis: description of the age-weight test and implications for further diagnostic investigation *J Pediatr Orthop.* 2001;21:481–487.
19. Rappaport EB, Fife D. Slipped capital femoral epiphysis in growth hormone-deficient patients. *Am J Dis Child.* 1985;139:369.
20. Grumbach MM, Bin-Abbas BS, Kaplan SL. The growth hormone cascade: progress and long-term results of growth hormone treatment in growth hormone deficiency. *Horm Res.* 1998;49(Suppl 2): 41–57.
21. Jingush S, Hara T, Sugioka Y. Deficiency of a parathyroid hormone fragment containing the midportion and 1,25-dihydroxyvitamin D in serum of patients with slipped capital femoral epiphysis. *J Pediatr Orthop.* 1997;17:216–219.
22. Rennie AM. Familial slipped upper femoral epiphysis. *J Bone Joint Surg Br.* 1967;49(3):535–539.
23. Manoff EM, Banffy MB, Winell JJ. Relationship between body mass index and slipped capital epiphysis. *J Pediatr Orthop.* 2005;25(6):744–746.
24. Loder RT, Aronson DD, Greenfield ML. The epidemiology of bilateral slipped capital femoral epiphysis. A study of children in Michigan. *J Bone Joint Surg Am.* 1993;75(8):1141–1147.
25. Puylaert D, Dimeglio A, Bentahur T. Staging puberty in slipped capital femoral epiphysis: importance of the triradiate cartilage. *J Pediatr Orthop.* 2004;24(2):144–147.
26. Poussa M, Schlenzka D, Yrjonen T. Body mass index and slipped capital femoral epiphysis. *J Pediatr Orthop B.* 2003;12:369–371.
27. Noguchi Y, Sakamaki T, and the Multicenter Study Committee of the Japanese Paediatric Orthopedic Association. Epidemiology and demographics of slipped capital femoral epiphysis in Japan: a multicenter study by the Japanese Paediatric Orthopaedic Association. *J Orthop Sci.* 2002;7:610–617.
28. Loder RT, Wittenberg B, DeSilva G. Slipped capital femoral epiphysis associated with endocrine disorders *J Pediatr Orthop.* 1995;15(3):349–356.
29. Mooney JF, Sanders JO, Browne RH, Anderson DJ, Jofe M, Feldman D, Raney EM. Management of unstable/acute slipped capital femoral epiphysis. Results of a Survey of the POSNA Membership. *J Pediatr Orthop.* 2005;25(2):162–166.

30. Leet AI, Skaggs DL. Evaluation of the acutely limping child. *Am Fam Physician.* 2000;61(4): 1011–1018.
31. Kocher MS, Bishop JA, Weed B, Hresko MT, Millis MB, Kim YJ, Kasser JR. Delay in diagnosis of slipped capital femoral epiphysis. *Pediatrics.* 2004;113:e322–325.
32. Uglow MG, Clarke NMP. The management of slipped capital femoral epiphysis. *J Bone Joint Surg Br.* 2004;86:631–635.
33. Loder RT. Slipped capital femoral epiphysis *Am Fam Physician.* 1998;57(9):2135–2142, 2148–2150.
34. Billing L, Bogren HG, Wallin J. Reliable X-ray diagnosis of slipped capital femoral epiphysis by combining the conventional and a new simplified geometrical method. *Pediatr Radiol.* 2002;32(6):423–430.
35. Umans H, Liebling MS, Moy L, Haramati N, Macy NJ, Pritzker HA. Slipped capital femoral epiphysis: a physeal lesion diagnosed by MRI, with radiographic and CT correlation. *Skeletal Radiol.* 1998;27(3):139–144.
36. Ballard J, Cosgrove AP. Anterior physeal separation: a sign indicating a high risk for avascular necrosis after slipped capital femoral epiphysis. *J Bone Joint Surg Br.* 2002;84(8):1176–1179.
37. Jofe MH, Lehman W, Ehrlich MG. Chondrolysis following a slipped capital femoral epiphysis. *J Pediatr Orthop.* 2004;13(1):29–31.
38. Eisenstein A, Rothschild S. Biochemical abnormalities in patients with slipped capital femoral epiphysis and chondrolysis. *J Bone Joint Surg.* 1976;58:459–467.
39. Givon U, Bowen JR. Chronic slipped capital femoral epiphysis: treatment by pinning in situ. *J Pediatr Orthop B.* 1999;8(3):216–222.
39a. Mullins MM, Sood M, Hashemi-Nejad A, Catterall A. The management of avascular necrosis after slipped capital femoral epiphysis. *J Bone Joint Surg Br.* 2005;87(12);1669–1674.
40. Langenskiold A. Tibia vara. A critical review. *Clin Orthop Relat Res.* 1989;246:195–207.
41. Davids JR, Huskamp M, Bagley AM. A dynamic biomechanical analysis of the etiology of adolescent tibia vara. *J Pediatr Orthop.* 1996;16:461–468.
42. Timm NL, Grupp-Phelan J, Ho ML. Chronic ankle morbidity in obese children following an acute ankle injury. *Arch Pediatr Adolesc Med.* 2005;159:33–36.
43. Song KM, Halliday S, Reilly C, Keezel W. Gait abnormalities following slipped capital femoral epiphysis. *J Pediatr Orthop.* 2004;24:148–154.

10

Gastrointestinal Complications

OVERVIEW

State of the Problem

One of the most problematic comorbidities of obesity is the spectrum of disease known as nonalcoholic fatty liver disease (NAFLD).

The association between obesity and steatosis, inflammation, and fibrosis was first noted in 1958 (1). However, the *impact* of this finding was not recognized until obesity became epidemic in the adult and child populations. NAFLD describes a continuum of conditions that range from simple steatosis at one end of the spectrum, through nonalcoholic steatohepatitis (NASH), to cirrhosis and end-stage liver disease (2).

The presence of hepatic steatosis in the general population has been estimated to be between 10% and 25%, making it the most common liver disease in developed countries (3). The prevalence of NAFLD is predicted to rise, driven by the increases in obesity, insulin resistance, and diabetes, the major risk factors for the disease.

The natural history of progression from NAFLD through NASH to cirrhosis is not well delineated, particularly in childhood. In some adult series, fibrosis and even cirrhosis are present in 15% to 50% of patients on initial biopsy (4). In a retrospective study of liver biopsies in pediatric patients believed to have NASH, some degree of fibrosis was present at the time of biopsy in 14 of 14 specimens (5). In a prospective study, 24 obese pediatric patients with NASH had liver biopsies, 17 (71%) had fibrosis, and 1 child had cirrhosis at diagnosis (6).

The prevalence of NAFLD in adults is estimated to be as high as 23% (7), with estimates of NASH (presence of NAFLD with inflammation and hepatocellular necrosis) in the adult population ranging between 1% and 3% (8) and 18.5% in obese adults (9). Liver disease in obese children and adolescents is largely a *silent* disease, usually discovered incidentally or on screening with little in the way of signs and symptoms. Hepatic steatosis was found in 53% of obese children evaluated by ultrasonography, with elevations of liver enzymes in 25% (10). Data from the National Health and Nutrition Examination Survey III (NHANES III) (1988–1994) showed that overall, 6% of overweight adolescents and 10% of obese adolescents already had elevated alanine aminotransferase (ALT) levels (11), an indication of hepatic inflammation and possible NASH (6).

Most patients with NAFLD have insulin resistance. Components of the metabolic syndrome, obesity, diabetes, and hyperlipidemia, are associated with NASH. In one study, 87% of patients with NASH fulfilled the criteria for the metabolic syndrome (12), and in studies of adult diabetic patients, more than one quarter have been found to have NASH (13). Type 2 diabetes, along with a higher body mass index (BMI), has also been associated with a greater rate of progression of fibrosis (14). When placed in the context of the escalating obesity epidemic and the increase in type 2 diabetes, the impact of this disease on affected children and adolescents is enormous.

Definitions

- **Hepatic steatosis**—Fatty deposition in hepatocytes.
- **Nonalcoholic fatty liver disease**—A continuum of conditions that range from simple steatosis to nonalcoholic steatohepatitis to cirrhosis and end-stage liver disease (2).
- **Nonalcoholic steatohepatitis (NASH)**—A liver disease characterized by steatosis (macrovesicular more than microvesciular), mixed mild lobular inflammation, presence of inflammatory cells, and hepatocellular ballooning in the absence of alcohol use; may include perisinusoidal fibrosis and Mallory bodies (15).

Etiology

The term NASH was first used by Ludwig and colleagues to describe hepatic histology consistent with alcoholic hepatitis in a group of obese, diabetic women who denied alcohol use (16,17).

The evolution of NASH is thought to be a two-stage process (18). The "first hit" is accumulation of fat in the liver, and the "second hit" is believed to involve increasing oxidative stress, which acts as a catalyst for the progression of simple steatosis to NASH (19). Free fatty acids (FFAs) accumulate within the hepatocytes and undergo oxidation, generating reactive oxygen species, which can react to form peroxides; the peroxides then cause membrane injury and release of tumor necrosis factor-α (TNF-α), which ultimately stimulates fibrosis (19) (Fig. 10.1).

Macrovesicular fat accumulates in the liver of patients with obesity and results from a combination of the following:

- Increased delivery
- Inadequate oxidation
- Decreased secretion of lipid out of the liver (15)

In a study of 144 adult patients (20), NASH was diagnosed by a persistent elevation of transaminases for more than 3 months, liver biopsy specimen with greater
than 10% fat, lobular and/or portal inflammation and/or Mallory bodies, fibrosis, or
cirrhosis with exclusion of other liver disease. In these adults, 26% had inflammation without abnormal fibrosis, 57% had some degree of fibrosis, and 17% had cirrhosis (20).

Most of our knowledge of the natural history of NAFLD and NASH comes from
adult studies. Steatosis without inflammation or fibrosis has been followed up in
adult patients for up to 16 years with no progression to cirrhosis (21). No similar
study has been performed in children. There is, however, controversy over whether
steatosis is a benign process.

NAFLD and NASH may be completely asymptomatic. In a series of adult patients
with the metabolic syndrome but normal liver enzymes, positive findings of NASH
were noted in 58 of 80 patients, 26 of 80 patients had fibrosis, and 8 of 80 patients
had silent cirrhosis. Risk factors for fibrosis were female gender, long history of
obesity, metabolic syndrome, and BMI greater than 45 (22).

Progression to NASH involves the development of inflammation and fibrosis, the
suggested second hit. Elevation of liver transaminases is taken as an indication of
inflammation, but fibrosis can be detected only by liver biopsy.

In one study, elevated ALT, hypertension, and insulin resistance were predictors
of NASH in severely obese adults undergoing obesity surgery (23). Fifty percent of
the patients identified with NASH also had diabetes. In those with diabetes, only 6%

NAFLD to NASH

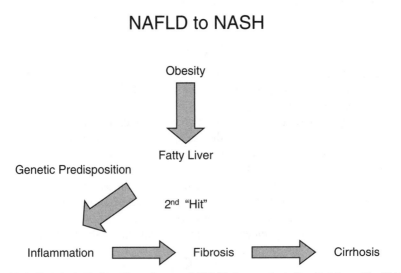

FIG. 10.1. Nonalcoholic fatty liver disease (NAFLD) to nonalcoholic steatohepatitis (NASH).
(Reprinted from Day CP, James OF. Steatohepatitis: a tale of two "hits"? *Gastroenterology.*
1998;114:842–845, with permission.)

had no evidence of NASH (23). Independent predictors of fibrosis in adult patients with NASH include age (>45 years), BMI greater than 31, and type 2 diabetes. An aspartate aminotransferase (AST)/ALT ratio of greater than 1 was associated with more severe fibrosis (20).

Hepatocellular necrosis on biopsy has been found to be a poor prognostic sign. In a series of 98 adults who were followed up for 10 years, 21% of patients with fat and ballooning degeneration and 28% of patients with fat and fibrosis developed cirrhosis compared with 4% of patients with fatty liver alone (24).

Pathophysiology

First Hit

The first hit in the pathophysiology of NAFLD is the accumulation of fat in the hepatocyte. In the presence of hyperinsulinemia, the adipocyte responds by increasing lipolysis and FFA delivery to the liver. Higher levels of insulin also prompt the hepatocytes to increase fatty acid synthesis and decrease fatty acid oxidation. There also may be increased degradation of apolipoprotein B 100, which is responsible for transporting excess FFAs out of the liver. All of these responses increase fat accumulation in the hepatocyte. Peripheral and hepatic insulin resistance has been found in almost all patients with NAFLD, irrespective of the coexistence of impaired glucose tolerance or obesity. Individuals with NAFD show impaired insulin-mediated suppression of hepatic glucose production compared with controls (12,25). Insulin resistance is significantly more common in patients with NASH than in those with other causes of noncirrhotic chronic liver disease (12). In a retrospective review of patients diagnosed with NASH, 18% of patients had an affected first-degree relative, suggesting the contribution of an inherited defect (26).

Second Hit

Fatty livers are unusually vulnerable to injury (17) and at increased risk for damage from other factors such as viruses, endotoxin, alcohol, and toxins (27). Multiple factors have been associated with the second hit, triggering the progression from steatosis to NASH. These include the following (18,19):

- Oxidative stress
- Depletion of important nutrients
- Cytokine upregulation
- Kupffer cell dysfunction
- Mitochondrial dysfunction
- Genetic predisposition
- Impaired hepatocyte regenerative processes
- Stellate cell activation (18,19)

Age is also a risk factor for cirrhosis, which may reflect the longer duration of risk for the second hit (20). Compared with controls, patients with NASH have increased expression of TNF-α messenger ribonucleic acid (mRNA) in liver and adipose tissue. The degree of overexpression correlates with histologic severity (28). TNF-α and endotoxin activate stellate cells, which increases collagen type I, the major collagen in fibrotic hepatic tissue (29). Higher serum TNF-α levels correlate with increased severity of NASH as manifested by greater inflammation and fibrosis (28).

NASH may be a recurring disease; fatty liver followed by steatohepatitis has been noted to develop after liver transplantation for cryptogenic cirrhosis (30). Leptin, which is present in elevated levels in obese individuals, promotes insulin resistance and in animal models alters insulin signaling in hepatocytes, resulting in increasing hepatocellular fatty acid production (31). Thus, elevated leptin levels occurring in obese patients may contribute to a metabolic environment that sustains hepatosteatosis.

Clinical Manifestations

Clinical symptoms of NASH, when they occur, are subtle and may include mild abdominal pain and fatigue. In adults, generalized fatigue, lethargy, and mild epigastric or right upper quadrant pain have been noted in 30% of patients (19).

If liver disease has progressed, patients may experience pruritus, anorexia, and nausea. When cirrhosis is present, patients may develop anasarca, variceal hemorrhage, and/or symptoms of hepatic failure (25). In a study of adults with NASH, obesity predicted progression of fibrosis, with one third having progression of fibrosis on a second biopsy 4 years after presentation. There were no differences between both groups regarding age, gender, diabetes, hyperlipidemia, ALT levels, AST-to-ALT ratio levels, albumin levels, prothrombin activity, steatosis, or inflammation (32). In a study of 310 obese children in Japan, 24% had an elevation in ALT. In a subgroup of 77 obese children with ALT values greater than 30 IU/L, 83% had a fatty liver on ultrasound compared with 18% of 27 children with normal ALT levels (33). Other factors associated with elevated ALT levels in overweight and obese adolescents include increased age, elevated glycosylated hemoglobin, elevated triglycerides, and decreased levels of serum antioxidants—vitamin E, β-carotene, and vitamin C (11).

In a series of 36 children, seen between 1985 and 1995, who presented with unexplained liver enzyme elevations to a gastroenterology clinic, 30 of the 36 patients were obese, 16 had hepatomegaly, and 13 had acanthosis nigricans. The mean value of AST was 104 ± 16 U/L (normal <37 U/L; range 26–523 U/L); the mean ALT value was 179 ± 31 U/L (normal <40 U/L; range 10–644 U/L). Liver ultrasound was performed in the majority of patients and showed increased echogenicity suggestive of fatty infiltration. There was no correlation between the severity of obesity and liver transaminase elevations. Biopsy was obtained in 24 of 36 patients. On biopsy, all children had large droplet (macrovesicular) steatosis, 21 children (88%) had inflammation, and 17 children (71%) had fibrosis. Fibrosis was moderately severe in 7 children and occurred in 2 children without evidence of inflammation (6). In a study of 228 obese children in Japan, hyperinsulinemia was correlated with NASH (34).

Evaluation

All obese children and adolescents should be evaluated for NASH.

Hepatic steatosis is prevalent in the obese population. A finding highly suggestive of hepatic steatosis on physical examination is hepatomegaly; however, this can sometimes be difficult to detect because of the degree of obesity. In addition, the finding of acanthosis nigricans should increase one's suspicion that the child may be at risk for hepatic steatosis. Liver ultrasound is the modality most commonly used for detecting hepatic steatosis. Computed tomography (CT) and magnetic resonance imaging (MRI) are also able to detect hepatic steatosis, although these modalities are more expensive and the CT scan unnecessarily exposes the patient to radiation. The diagnosis of NAFLD can be made in the presence of hepatic steatosis after other causes of fatty liver are excluded (Table 10.1). Tests of liver inflammation should be performed and include AST, ALT, and γ-glutamyltransferase (GGT). Tests for alkaline phosphatase (ALK PO4), total bilirubin, and albumin can also be considered. Other

TABLE 10.1. *Differential diagnosis of hepatic steatosis*

Nutritional stress	**Chemotherapeutic agents**
Systemic disease	Methotrexate
Malnutrition	Prednisone/Prednisolone
Total parenteral nutrition	L-asparaginase
Inflammatory bowel disease	Tomoxifen
Celiac disease	**Hepatotoxic drugs**
Liver-based metabolic disease	Zidovudine and anti-HIV treatments
Mauriac's syndrome	Ethanol
Alpha$_1$-antitrypsin deficiency	Ecstasy
Wilson's disease	Hypervitaminosis A
Schwachman's syndrome	Valproate
Glycogen storage disease	Amiodarone
Disorders of fatty acid beta-oxidation	**Infections**
Mitochondrial and peroxisomal defects	Hepatitis C
of fatty acid oxidation	Hepatitis B
Disorders of adipose tissue	**Other**
Lipodystrophies	Weber-Christian disease
Inherited enzyme deficiencies	Cystic fibrosis
Abetalipoproteinemia	Cobalamin C disease
Galactosemia	
Fructosemia	
Wolman's disease (cholesterol ester	
storage disease)	
Carbamoyl phosphate synthetase deficiency	
Long chain fatty acyl dehydrogenase	
deficiency	

Data from Baldridge AD, Perez-Atayde AR, Graeme-Cook F, Higgins L, Lavine J. Idiopathic steatohepatitis in childhood: a multicenter retrospective study. *J Pediatr.* 1995;127:700–704; Marion AW, Baker AJ, Dharwan A. Fatty liver disease in children. *Arch Dis Child.* 2004;89:648–652.

causes of liver inflammation should be eliminated before making the diagnosis of NASH (Table 10.2).

> Liver biopsy remains essential for diagnosing and evaluating the progression of NASH.

Imaging studies, as noted previously, are able to detect steatosis but are not accurate predictors of fibrosis. If the previously mentioned evaluation does not reveal a cause of elevated liver enzymes, a liver biopsy should be considered because this is

TABLE 10.2. *Evaluation of elevation of liver enzymes in obese children*

Nonspecific liver dysfunction
  AST, ALT
  Coagulation studies
  Total protein
  Albumin, lactate, pyruvate
NASH-associated metabolic abnormalities
  Glucose, glucose tolerance test
  Hyperinsulinemia, hyperlipidemia
Viral hepatitis
  Serology for hepatitis B surface antigen, antibody to hepatitis B surface antigen, antibody to hepatitis B core antigen, and hepatitis C antibodies, hepatitis C PCR (if indicated)
  HIV antibodies
  EBV antibodies
Autoimmune hepatitis
  Anti-smooth-muscle antibodies, anti-liver, kidney, microsomal antibody, ANA sedimentation rate, CF alleles, immunoglobulin G, or total immunoglobulins
  Nonspecific tissue antibodies
Drug-induced liver disease
  History of corticosteroid, high-dose estrogens, methotrexate, tetracycline, calcium channel blockers, amiodarone use
  Biliary cirrhosis/Biliary obstruction
  Bilirubin, direct and indirect
Wilson's disease
  Serum copper, ceruloplasmin, 24-hour urinary copper
Alcoholic liver disease
  Random ethanol level
Alpha$_1$-antitrypsin deficiency
  Alpha$_1$-antitrypsin level and phenotype
Hemochromatosis
  Iron, ferritin, total iron binding capacity (genetic testing for hemochromatosis can then be considered if the above are suggestive of hemochromatosis)

AST, aspartate aminotransferase; ALT, alanine aminotransferase; NASH, nonalcoholic steatohepatitis; PCR, polymerase chain reaction; HIV, human immunodeficiency virus; EBV, Epstein-Barr virus; ANA, antinuclear antibody; CF, cystic fibrosis.

Data from Baldridge AD, Perez-Atayde AR, Graeme-Cook F, Higgins L, Lavine J. Idiopathic steatohepatitis in childhood: a multicenter retrospective study. *J Pediatr.* 1995;127:700–704; Marion AW, Baker AJ, Dharwan A. Fatty liver disease in children. *Arch Dis Child.* 2004;89:648–652; Lavine JE. Vitamin E treatment of nonalcoholic steatohepatitis in children: a pilot study. *J Pediatr.* 2000;136:734–738.

the most accurate means of truly assessing the degree of inflammation and fibrosis, which is essential for making a definitive diagnosis and evaluating the prognosis of NASH.

Indications for liver biopsy are not standardized in adults and are even more problematic in children and adolescents. Day (35) lists some indicators for deciding on biopsy in adults:

1. ALT greater than twice the normal value
2. AST greater than ALT
3. Moderate "central" obesity
4. Impaired glucose tolerance or diabetes
5. Hypertension
6. Hypertriglyceridemia.

Biopsy findings of NASH include steatosis, predominantly macrosteatosis; ballooning of hepatocytes; perisinusoidal fibrosis; and mixed lobular inflammatory infiltrate (36).

The classification of NAFLD and NASH is histopathologic and is outlined in Table 10.3. The histologic appearance of NASH is illustrated in Figures 10.2, 10.3, and 10.4.

Treatment

There is no single standardized treatment for patients with NAFLD or NASH. The treatment of NAFLD should focus on preventing or reversing events that provoke inflammation and insulin resistance.

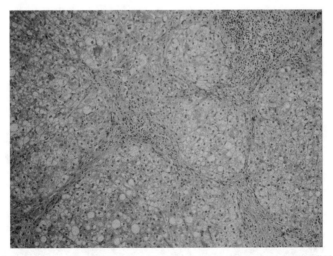

FIG. 10.2. A liver biopsy from a 10-year-old with nonalcoholic steatohepatitis (NASH) shows fatty infiltration (clear) with intrahepatocellular fat, portal inflammation, and bridging fibrosis.

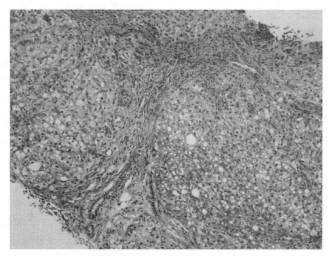

FIG. 10.3. A higher magnification view of extensive bridging fibrosis.

Because of the association of NASH with obesity, weight loss has been a mainstay of treatment. Early studies of adult postsurgical bariatric patients showed that *drastic* weight loss could lead to increased inflammation and fibrosis. This was thought to be due to increased production of FFAs and lipid peroxidation increasing oxidative stress. This finding has led to caution and a recommendation to avoid rapid weight loss in these patients (37). Gradual weight loss and control of diabetes will reduce hepatosteatosis as well as transaminase elevation (38,39).

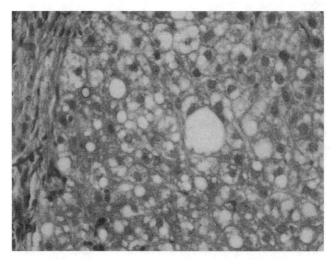

FIG. 10.4. High-power view of panacinar steatosis.

TABLE 10.3. *Brunt Classification of nonalcoholic fatty liver disease*

Macrovesicular steatosis
Grade 0: None
Grade 1: <33% of liver involved with steatosis
Grade 2: 33%–66% of liver involved with steatosis
Grade 3: > 66% of liver involved steatosis
Necroinflammatory activity
Grade 1 (mild): steatosis <66%, occasional ballooned hepatocyte (zone 3), scattered intra-acinar neutrophils (PMNs ± lymphocytes), no or mild portal inflammation
Grade 2 (moderate): steatosis of any degree, obvious zone 3 ballooning degeneration, intra-acinar PMNs, zone 3 perisinusoidal fibrosis may be present, mild-to-moderate, portal and intra-acinar inflammation
Grade 3 (severe): panacinar steatosis, widespread ballooning and intra-acinar inflammation, PMNs associated with ballooned hepatocytes, mild to moderate portal inflammation
Staging of NAFLD
Stage 1: Zone 3 perisinusoidal/pericellular fibrosis, focally or extensively present
Stage 2: Zone 3 perisinusoidal/pericellular fibrosis with focal or extensive periportal fibrosis
Stage 3: Zone 3 perisinusoidal/pericellular fibrosis and portal fibrosis with focal or extensive bridging fibrosis
Stage 4: Cirrhosis

NAFLD, nonalcoholic fatty liver disease; PMNs, polymorphonuclear leukocytes.
Data from Poordad FF. Nonalcoholic fatty liver disease: a review. *Expert Opin Emerging Drugs.* 2005;10:661–670; Brunt EM, Janney CG, Di Bisceglie AM, Neuschwander-Tetri BA, Bacon BR. Nonalcoholic steatohepatitis: a proposal for grading and staging the histological lesions. *Am J Gastroenterol.* 1999;94:2467–2474.

In a small study of adults who used diet and exercise to reduce weight over a 3-month period, liver enzymes improved, as did liver histology, compared with no change in the control group (40). In another series of adults who underwent adjustable gastric band placement and weight loss, there were improvements in lobular steatosis, necroinflammatory changes, and fibrosis on a second biopsy 2 years after surgery. This improvement was more pronounced in patients with characteristics of the metabolic syndrome who had been more severely affected prior to surgery (41). In a small series of pediatric patients with elevated aminotransferases and fatty liver on ultrasound, those who lost at least 10% of their excess weight showed normalized ALT and AST values and decreased ultrasound evidence of fatty infiltration (39). In another series of obese children who underwent ultrasonography at the start of a diet and exercise program, 53% had evidence of liver steatosis noted on ultrasound and 25% had elevated transaminase values. Both steatosis and liver enzyme elevations resolved with weight loss (10).

Orlistat, a gastric and pancreatic lipase inhibitor, has been studied in small groups of adult patients as a treatment for NASH. In one study of 10 obese adults with biopsy-proven NASH, treatment with orlistat and dietary counseling for 6 months improved steatosis in more than one half and fibrosis in one third of the patients (42). No similar studies have been performed in children.

Metformin has been tried in the treatment of NASH in adults and, despite improvements in insulin resistance and a decrease in liver enzymes, there was no significant change in inflammation or fibrosis when compared with patients with NASH who underwent dietary treatment alone (43).

Treatment of NASH with peroxisome proliferator activated receptor agonists (thiazolidinediones) remains experimental and has been tried in adults. These drugs have not been tested in children. The initial studies were carried out with troglitazone, which has been withdrawn from the market because of hepatotoxicity. Improvement in steatosis, cellular injury, parenchymal inflammation, and fibrosis has been seen with rosiglitazone; however, weight gain and increased liver enzymes occurred after treatment (44).

Because oxidative stress is considered to play a role in the etiology of NASH, antioxidants such as vitamin E have been used in treatment. Results have been disappointing, with most studies showing no or only minor improvement in inflammation and fibrosis (45). A pediatric study using vitamin E showed normalization of liver enzymes but did not include liver biopsy in the study (46).

Currently, treatment of NASH in children should center on a nutrition and exercise plan to promote gradual weight loss, treatment of diabetes if present, and avoidance of other agents that are hepatotoxic. Orlistat is approved for weight loss in children but has not been evaluated in the pediatric age group for treatment of NASH. Inhibition of fibrosis remains a target of therapy for NASH, but no drugs are yet approved as antifibrotic drugs in humans.

Alcohol intake is associated with severe liver disease in obese adults (47). In one study, approximately 50% of obese adolescents who reported modest alcohol ingestion (four times per month or more) had elevated ALT levels (11). Ethanol has been found to induce cytochrome P450, which is responsible for activating metabolites to toxic intermediaries and is already increased in patients with NASH. There is concern about further insult to the liver in children with NASH, and agents associated with liver toxicity, especially alcohol, should be avoided.

Summary

All children with BMI greater than the 95th percentile should be screened for NASH with liver inflammation studies (ALT, AST, GGT). Children with elevated transaminases should have a thorough evaluation to rule out other causes of liver disease. Ultrasound may be performed to document steatosis. Children should be evaluated for diabetes and impaired glucose tolerance, which should be addressed if necessary, as well as for other components of the metabolic syndrome (i.e., hypertension, hyperlipidemia, elevated waist/hip ratio). Assessment for any additional obesity-related comorbidities should be completed. Using lifestyle modifications of nutrition and physical activity, weight loss is an important goal. Liver biopsy should be considered to definitively determine diagnosis and evaluate for inflammation and fibrosis as a means of assessing severity and prognosis. If fibrosis is present, lifestyle intervention should be intensified and liver disease closely monitored, with consideration being given to enrollment in promising therapeutic trials if available.

SPECIAL SITUATIONS

Hypothalamic and Pituitary Disease

> Patients who have hypothalamic and/or pituitary dysfunction may be at increased risk for NAFLD.

In one series of 21 patients with hypothalamic/pituitary dysfunction caused by brain tumor, idiopathic hypopituitarism (6/21), hypophysitis (1/21), and Prader-Willi syndrome (1/21), NAFLD was diagnosed within 6 years of diagnosis. In follow-up, 2 underwent liver transplant, and 1 died of hepatocellular carcinoma (48). Children with hypothalamic injury or disease should be evaluated and followed up for the development of NAFLD and NASH; aggressive lifestyle therapy focusing on nutrition and activity should be pursued.

ONGOING SUPPORT: CASE OF MK

Initial Presentation

MK is a 13-year-old white boy who comes for a physical examination prior to playing fall sports. He is 5 ft 7 in. tall and weighs 195 lb, with a BMI of 30.5. His blood pressure is 123/78 mm Hg. He has had no serious illnesses since he was last seen 1 year ago. He has had some minor complaints of intermittent nausea and occasional headaches. He is not taking any medication. He has done well in school and participates in several sports. His parents are both overweight, and his maternal grandfather has just been diagnosed with type 2 diabetes and hypertension.

You perform a review of systems, paying particular attention to obesity-related comorbidities. He is having occasional headaches, which are self-limited, and he reports no difficulties with vision. He denies shortness of breath, wheezing, snoring, restless sleeping, or daytime tiredness. He does have some nausea, which he attributes to "what I ate." He is not complaining of any hip or knee pain. He reports he is "feeling good" and has not been sad or unhappy. On physical examination you note that his blood pressure is slightly elevated, he has centripetal obesity, and he has mild acanthosis nigricans of his neck and axilla. He is Tanner stage III. Because he meets the criteria of obesity/overweight for an adolescent (BMI is at the 95th percentile for age and gender), you screen for obesity-related comorbidities with laboratory studies. You let MK and his mother know that you are ordering laboratory studies for diabetes and for dyslipidemia and liver disease.

You begin your discussion with MK and his mother by showing them his growth chart and BMI. Mrs. K comments that MK is a "big boy" just like the rest of the family and says that his weight does not worry her. MK denies any concern about his weight but does say that he wishes he could run a little faster. You review the family history and note that not only his maternal grandmother but also several aunts and uncles have hypertension and diabetes; his mother says that MK's doctor had just mentioned that he had "borderline" diabetes at his last physical. You mention that MK has slightly elevated blood pressure and acanthosis nigricans and discuss these findings in light of the family history and the risk of type 2 diabetes. Mrs. K says that the family "should probably do something about it."

With this lead you ask MK to review his daily eating and activity with you. He notes he is skipping breakfast, eating a school lunch, buying a soda and chips after school, and eating one to two portions of dinner. The family eats out two or three times per week, and Mrs. K notes that MK often brings snacks to his room after dinner to eat while playing computer games. MK estimates that he is drinking about five regular sodas per day. When you ask about screen time, Mrs. K gives a pointed look at MK and says, "he is playing on the computer all the time." MK says that besides his 1 hour of homework, he plays on the computer from the time he gets home from school or sports until bedtime. You estimate about 4 to 5 hours per day.

You explain to MK and his mother that the five sodas a day that he is drinking represent about 750 kcal, the equivalent of 50 teaspoons of sugar. His mother is surprised and expresses willingness to buy water and diet soda for the family instead. MK shrugs and says that drinking diet instead of regular soda "would be ok." You agree with his mother that this is a good place to start, and you schedule a follow-up visit to review test results and note progress on the change from regular soda.

Three Weeks Later

When MK returns in 3 weeks, you note that his weight is 192 lb, his height is 5 ft 7 in., and his BMI is 30.1. His blood pressure is 119/76 mm Hg. He and his mother report that the family is now drinking diet drinks or water between meals; MK says he has a regular soda "once in a while," usually when he is with his friends. You congratulate them on making this important change and review the results of the laboratory tests with them (Table 10.4).

You begin by explaining that MK's elevated fasting insulin indicates insulin resistance and places him in the continuum of risk for type 2 diabetes, especially coupled with his high BMI, acanthosis nigricans, and positive family history. You note that the high values of cholesterol and especially triglycerides often accompany insulin elevations. In addition to these findings, his liver enzymes are elevated, which indi-

TABLE 10.4. *Case study laboratory test results*

Fasting glucose, 96 mg/dL	GGT, 56 U/L
AST, 93 U/L[a]	Total cholesterol, 175 mg/dL[a]
HgbA$_{1C}$, 5.8%	HDL cholesterol, 36 mg/dL[a]
ALT, 76 U/L[a]	Triglycerides, 215 mg/dL[a]
Fasting insulin, 40 µU/mL[a]	

AST, aspartate aminotransferase; ALT, alanine aminotransferase; GGT, γ-glutamyltransferase; HDL, high-density lipoprotein.
[a]Abnormal values.

cate inflammation in his liver, possibly due to fatty infiltration. This alarms his mother because she never realized the liver could be affected by his weight gain.

Next Steps

In consultation with a pediatric gastroenterologist, you order laboratory studies to rule out other causes of liver disease (Table 10.2) and order a liver ultrasound to detect fatty infiltration. You discuss liver biopsy, but the gastroenterologist points out that there are currently no pediatric criteria for biopsy (studies are in progress) and MK does not meet the adult criteria. You decide to pursue the laboratory work and ultrasound while you are working with MK and his family on a weight loss plan.

You explain your discussion with the pediatric gastroenterologist, the fact that you are ordering laboratory tests to rule out other causes of liver problems and an ultrasound of the liver. You emphasize that the only known treatment for NASH is weight loss and let MK and his mother know they have made a good start and you will be working with them to continue the process of change. You suggest that they may want to consider another change in eating and activity to decrease MK's energy intake. Together you, MK, and his mother decide that reducing the number of times he and the family eat out and substituting healthy snacks would be the next step. You also work with MK on a plan to exercise on the days he does not have sports practice and to try cut back 1 hour on his computer use.

You review the diagnostic and treatment plan and also caution MK that certain medications have liver-related side effects and he should check with you before taking any new medicine; emphasize that this is an additional reason not to drink alcohol.

You plan to see MK monthly to check on his weight and lifestyle changes, as well as to keep him updated on new diagnosis and treatment data from studies of NASH as they are completed.

REFERENCES

1. Westwater JO, Fainer D. Liver impairment in the obese. *Gastroenterology.* 1958;34:686–693.
2. Harrison SA, Diehl AM. Fat and the liver—a molecular overview. *Semin Gastrointest Dis.* 2002; 13:3–16.
3. Poordad FF. Nonalcoholic fatty liver disease: a review. *Expert Opin Emerging Drugs.* 2005; 10:661–670.
4. James OF, Day CP. Nonalcoholic steatohepatitis (NASH): a disease of emerging identity and importance. *J Hepatol.* 1998;29(3):495–501.
5. Baldridge AD, Perez-Atayde AR, Graeme-Cook F, Higgins L, Lavine JE. Idiopathic steatohepatitis in childhood: a multicenter retrospective study. *J Pediatr.* 1995;127(5):700–704.
6. Rashid M, Roberts EA. Nonalcoholic steatohepatitis in children. *J Pediatr Gastroenterol Nutr.* 2000;30:48–53.
7. Clark JM, Brancati FL, Diehl AM. Nonalcoholic fatty liver disease. *Gastroenterology.* 2002;122(6): 1649–1657.
8. Angulo P. Nonalcoholic fatty liver disease. *N Engl J Med.* 2002;346(16):1221–1231.
9. Wanless IR, Lentz JS. Fatty liver hepatitis (steatohepatitis) and obesity: an autopsy study with analysis of risk factors. *Hepatology.* 1990;12(5):1106–1110.
10. Franzese A, Vajro P, Argenziano A, Puzziello A, Iannucci MP, Saviano MC, Brunetti M, Rubino A. Liver involvement in obese children. Ultrasonography and liver enzyme levels at diagnosing and during follow-up in an Italian population. *Dig Dis Sci.* 1997;42(7):1428–1442.

11. Strauss RS, Barlow SE, Dietz WH. Prevalence of abnormal serum aminotransferase values in overweight and obese adolescents. *J Pediatr.* 2000;136(6):727–733.
12. Chitturi S, Abeygunasekera S, Farrell GC, Holmes-Walker J, Hui JM, Fung C, Karim R, Lin R, Samarasinghe D, Liddle C, Weltman M, George J. NASH and insulin resistance: insulin hypersecretion and specific association with the insulin residence syndrome. *Hepatology.* 2002;35(2):373–379.
13. Gupte P, Amarapurkar D, Agal S, Baijal R, Kulshrestha P, Pramanik S, Patel N, Madan A, Amarapurkar A, Hafeezunnisa. Non-alcoholic steatohepatitis in type 2 diabetes mellitus. *J Gastroenterol Hepatol.* 2004;19:854–858.
14. Adams LA, Sanderson S, Lindor KD, Angulo P. The histological course of nonalcoholic fatty liver disease: a longitudinal study of 103 patients with sequential liver biopsies. *J Hepatol.* 2005;42(1): 132–138.
15. Brunt EM. Nonalcoholic steatohepatitis: definition and pathology. *Semin Liver Dis.* 2001;21:3–16.
16. Ludwig J, Viggiano TR, McGill DB, Oh BJ. Nonalcoholic steatohepatitis: Mayo Clinic experiences with a hitherto unnamed disease. *Mayo Clin Proc.* 1980;55(7):434–438.
17. McCullough AJ. Update on nonalcoholic fatty liver disease. *J Clin Gastroenterol.* 2002;34(3): 255–262.
18. Day CP, James OF. Steatohepatitis: a tale of two "hits"? *Gastroenterology.* 1998;114(4):842–845.
19. Harrison SA, Kadakia S, Lang KA, Schenker S. Nonalcoholic steatohepatitis: what we know in the new millennium. *Am J Gastroenterol.* 2002;97:2714–2724.
20. Angulo P, Keach JC, Batts KP, Lindor KD. Independent predictors of liver fibrosis in patient with nonalcoholic steatohepatitis. *Hepatology.* 1999;30(6):1356–1362.
21. Teli MR, James OF, Burt AD, Bennett MK, Day CP. The natural history of nonalcoholic fatty liver: a follow-up study. *Hepatology.* 1995;22:1714–1719.
22. Sorrentino P, Tarantino G, Conca P, Perrella A, Terracciano ML, Vecchione R, Gargiulo G, Gennarelli N, Lobello R. Silent non-alcoholic fatty liver disease—a clinical-histological study. *J Hepatol.* 2004;41(5):751–757.
23. Dixon JB, Bhathal PS, O'Brian PE. Nonalcoholic fatty liver disease: predictors of nonalcoholic steatohepatitis and liver fibrosis in the severely obese. *Gastroenterology.* 2001;121:91–100.
24. Matteoni CA, Younossi ZM, Gramlich T, Boparai N, Liu YC, McCullough AJ. Nonalcoholic fatty liver disease: a spectrum of clinical and pathological severity. *Gastroenterology.* 1999;116: 1413–1419.
25. Contos MJ, Sanyal AJ. The clinicopathologic spectrum and management of nonalcoholic fatty liver disease. *Adv Anat Pathol.* 2002;9:37–51.
26. Willner IR, Waters B, Patil SR, Reuben A, Morelli J, Riely C A. Ninety patients with nonalcoholic steatohepatitis:insulin resistance, familial tendency, and severity of disease. *Am J Gastroenterol.* 2001;96:2957–2961.
27. Yang SO, Lin HZ, Loane MD, Clemens M, Diehl AM. Obesity increases sensitivity to endotoxin liver injury: implications for the pathogenesis of steatohepatitis. *Proc Natl Acad Sci U S A.* 1997; 94(6):2557–2562.
28. Crespo J, Cayon A, Fernandez-Gil P, Hernandez-Guerra M, Mayorga M, Dominguez-Diez A, Fernandez-Escalante JC, Pons-Romero F. Gene expression of tumor necrosis factor alpha and TNF receptors p55 and p57 in nonalcoholic steatohepatitis patients. *Hepatology.* 2001;34:1158–1163.
29. Lee KS, Buck M, Houglum K, Chojkier M. Activation of hepatic stellate cells by TGF alpha and collagen type I is mediated by oxidative stress through c-myb expression. *J Clin Invest.* 1995;96: 2461–2468.
30. Contos MJ, Cales W, Sterling RK, Luketic VA, Shiffman ML, Mills AS, Fisher RA, Ham J, Sanyal AJ. Development of nonalcoholic fatty liver disease after orthotopic liver transplant for cryptogenic cirrhosis. *Liver Transpl.* 2001;7:363–373.
31. Koteish A, Diehl AM. Animal models of steatosis. *Semin Liver Dis.* 2001;21:89–101.
32. Fassio E, Alvarez E, Dominguez N, Landeira G, Long C. Natural history of nonalcoholic steatohepatitis: a longitudinal study of repeat liver biopsies. *Hepatology.* 2004;40(4):820–826.
33. Tazawa Y, Noguchi H, Nishinomiya F, Takada G. Serum alanine aminotransferase activity in obese children. *Acta Paediatr.* 1997;86:238–241.
34. Kawasaki T, Hashimoto N, Kikuchi T, Takahashi H, Uchiyama M. The relationship between fatty liver and hyperinsulinemia in obese Japanese children. *J Pediatr Gastroenterol Nutr.* 1997;24: 317–321.
35. Day CP. Nonalcoholic steatohepatitis (NASH); where are we now and where are we going? *Gut.* 2002;50(5):585–588.

36. Burt AD, Mutton A, Day C. Diagnosis and interpretation of steatosis and steatohepatitis. *Semin Diagn Pathol.* 1998;15:246–258.

37. Luyckx FH, Desaive C, Thiry A, Dewe W, Scheen AJ, Gielen JE, Lefebvre PJ. Liver abnormalities in severely obese subjects: effect of drastic weight loss after gastroplasty. *Int J Obes.* 1998;22:222–226.

38. Youseff W, McCullough AJ. Diabetes mellitus, obesity and hepatic steatosis. *Semin Gastrointestinal Dis.* 2002;13:17–30.

39. Vajro P, Fontanella A, Perna C, Orso G, Tadesco M, De Viscenco A. Persistent hyperaminotransferasemia resolving after weight reduction in obese children. *J Pediatr.* 1994;125(2):239–241.

40. Ueno T, Sugawara H, Sujaku K, Hashimoto O, Tsuji R, Tamaki S, Torimura T, Inuzuka S, Sata M, Tanikawa K. Therapeutic effects of restricted diet and exercise in obese patient with fatty liver. *J Hepatol.* 1997;27(1):103–107.

41. Dixon JB, Bhathal PS, Hughes NR, O'Brien PE. Nonalcoholic fatty liver disease: improvement in liver histological analysis with weight loss. *Hepatology.* 2004;39(6):1647–1654.

42. Harrison SA, Fincke C, Helinski D, Torgerson S, Hayashi P. A pilot study of orlistat treatment in obese, non-alcoholic steatohepatitis patients. *Aliment Pharmacol Ther.* 2004;20(6):623–628.

43. Uygun A, Kadayifci A, Isik AT, Ozgurtas T, Deveci S, Tuzun A, Yesilova Z, Gulsen M, Dagalp K. Metformin in the treatment of patients with nonalcoholic steatohepatitis. *Aliment Pharmacol Ther.* 2004;19(5):537–544.

44. Neuschwander-Tetri BA, Brunt EM, Wehmeier DR, Oliver D, Bacon BR. Improved nonalcoholic steatohepatitis after 48 weeks of treatment with the PPAR-gamma ligand rosiglitazone. *Hepatology.* 2003;38(4):1008-1017.

45. Adams LA, Angulo P. Vitamin E and C for the treatment of NASH duplication of results but lack of demonstration of efficacy. *Am J Gastroenterol.* 2003;98(11):2348–2350.

46. Lavine JE. Vitamin E treatment of nonalcoholic steatohepatitis in children: a pilot study. *J Pediatr.* 2000;136(6):734–738.

47. Naveau S, Giraud V, Borotto E, et al. Excess weight risk factor for alcoholic liver disease. *Hepatology.* 1997;25:108–111.

48. Adams LA, Feldstein A, Lindor KD, Angulo P. Nonalcoholic fatty liver disease among patients with hypothalamic and pituitary dysfunction. *Hepatology.* 2004;39(4):909–914.

11

Renal Complications

Adult obesity has been associated with an increase in end-stage renal disease (ESRD) (1). In a prospective study of adults 18 years and older, followed up for 15 to 35 years, elevated body mass index (BMI) at baseline was associated with a greater rate of ESRD, defined as disease requiring dialysis or renal transplantation (2). There was a 10-fold increase in ESRD between adults who were normal weight and those with morbid obesity (BMI ≥40). The risk for ESRD rose continuously with an increase in BMI. The relationship of ESRD to BMI persisted after controlling for gender, race, education level, smoking, diabetes, hypertension, and baseline renal disease (2). Microalbuminuria has also been associated with the development of early renal disease (3). Microalbuminuria is also considered an early indication of vascular damage, a precursor of atherosclerosis (4), and is associated with the development of cardiovascular disease (5).

ETIOLOGY

Obesity in adults can result in distinct glomerulopathology consisting of glomerulomegaly with or without segmental sclerosis (6). In adolescents, hypertrophy of the glomerulus, focal segmental glomerulosclerosis, and increased mesangial matrix and cellularity with preservation of foot process were found in a review of renal biopsies in obese adolescents with proteinuria and mild hypertension in the absence of inflammatory or immunologic changes (7).

Studies in obese adults have shown that cardiac output and expanded extracellular and intravascular volume increase the renal perfusion rate (8). In a study of obese and lean adults, glomerular filtration rate and effective renal plasma flow were higher in overweight than in normal weight patients (8). Urinary albumin excretion was higher in both obese normotensive and obese hypertensive patients than in their normal weight counterparts (8).

In obese Zucker rats, glomerular filtration rates are increased along with an expansion of glomerular area and mesangial matrix (9). Glomerular lesions in obese Zucker rats have been correlated with cholesterol levels, proteinuria, triglyceride levels, insulin levels, creatinine levels, and glucose levels. Histologically, glomerular damage involved early podocyte damage and tubulointerstitial injury. Use of an angiotensin-converting enzyme (ACE) inhibitor normalized proteinuria, cholesterol levels, glomerular lesions, and podocyte morphology (10).

Obese children have been found to have a higher urinary albumin/creatinine ratio and urinary β_2-microglobulin/creatinine ratio than normal weight children, possibly indicating early renal glomerular and tubular dysfunction. The urinary albumin/creatinine ratio was associated with fasting hyperinsulinemia, impaired glucose tolerance, and hypercholesterolemia and significantly correlated with fasting glucose and 2-hour glucose during a 2-hour plasma glucose tolerance test. Urinary albumin/creatinine ratios also increased in accordance with the number of features of the metabolic syndrome in these obese children (11).

Obesity has been shown to worsen renal failure in adults and is one of the treatment factors targeted to slow progression of renal failure.

A study of pediatric patients with chronic renal disease showed that an increase in obesity coincided with a significant rise in the incidence of chronic renal insufficiency (12).

Hormonal changes and low-grade inflammation associated with obesity have also been suggested as mechanisms responsible for obesity-related renal damage (13).

Increased synthesis of vasoactive and fibrogenic substances, including angiotensin II, insulin, leptin, and transforming growth factor–β (TGF-β), which are increased in obesity, may affect glomerular hyperfiltration, mesangial cell hypertrophy, and matrix production (14). Leptin, which is produced in adipose tissue and is cleared principally by the kidney, stimulates cellular proliferation, TGF-β_1 synthesis, and type IV collagen production in glomerular endothelial cells. In mesangial cells, leptin increases type I collagen production. Infusion of leptin into normal rats fostered the development of focal glomerulosclerosis and proteinuria. In addition, leptin has been shown to increase sodium excretion, increase sympathetic activity, and stimulate production of reactive oxygen species in the kidney, suggesting a direct pathophysiologic link between obesity and renal pathology (15).

Renal disease is one of the most serious complications of type 2 diabetes, and diabetic nephropathy secondary to type 2 diabetes is the most common cause of ESRD in adults (16).

The most characteristic renal lesion in diabetes is diffuse and nodular glomerulosclerosis (Kimmelstiel-Wilson lesion). Diffuse glomerulosclerosis was present in 65% of Pima Indians with type 2 diabetes on autopsy (17).

DEFINITIONS

- **Microalbuminuria**—The excretion of albumin greater than normal but less than the detection limits of urine dipstick methods, albuminuria 30 to 300 mg per 24 hours (15–200 μg/minute) (16,18). The simplest screening measure is a random urine microalbumin/creatinine ratio (μg/mg), which should be less than or equal to 30 μg/mg (19).
- **Proteinuria**—Glomerular proteinuria, which usually follows microalbuminuria, is an early sign of diabetic nephropathy (16). It is usually first evident as a dipstick urine protein value greater than or equal to 1+ (30 mg/dL). Proteinuria is defined as levels of protein excretion greater than 300 mg per 24 hours or a urinary total protein (mg/dL)/creatinine (mg/dL) ratio greater than 0.2 (16).

EVALUATION

The 24-hour urine collection is the standard measure of microalbuminuria. However, the use of microalbumin/creatinine ratio in a morning urine specimen is closely correlated with 24-hour albumin in adults (20).

CLINICAL MANIFESTATIONS

> Microalbuminuria can be considered a direct risk factor for progression of renal disease and an integrated risk marker for cardiovascular disease (20).

It is associated with hypertension, endothelial dysfunction, and hyperhomocysteinemia (20). Microalbuminuria is a marker for diabetic nephropathy in both type 1 and type 2 diabetes (18).

Diabetic nephropathy is similar in both type 1 and type 2 diabetes in adults and responds to glycemic control and treatment with ACE inhibitors. In adults with diabetes—and with hypertension and cardiovascular disease in first-degree relatives—glycemic control, hypertension, and smoking are predictors of nephropathy (21). Adults with type 1 and type 2 diabetes had similar rates of proteinuria after 20 years (27% and 28%, respectively). After 25 years of diabetes, these percentages increased to 46% in type 1 diabetes and 57% in type 2 diabetes. After 5 years of proteinuria, the rates of renal failure were 63% for type 2 diabetes and 59% for type 1 (22).

Poor glycemic control, lack of physical exercise, hypertension, heart failure, and nondiabetic renal disease can contribute to microalbuminuria. In adults with type 2 diabetes, proteinuria and microalbuminuria have been shown to predict subsequent clinical nephropathy and mortality from cardiovascular disease (16).

Microalbuminuria has been associated with increased cardiovascular mortality in adults without diabetes. Microalbuminuria was associated with impaired glucose tolerance and parental history of type 2 diabetes as well as a higher incidence of hypertension, decreased high-density lipoprotein (HDL) cholesterol, elevated triglycerides, and increased 2-hour insulin (23). The association between microalbuminuria and cardiovascular morbidity increased in a linear fashion with the degree of albumin excretion in adults (24). A link has also been found between urinary albumin excretion in adults and left ventricular hypertrophy (20).

Microalbuminuria has been detected in slightly more than 10% of a cohort of obese children with a BMI greater than the 97th percentile. The presence of microalbuminuria was associated with higher glucose and insulin levels during an oral glucose tolerance test independent of BMI, age, gender, ethnicity, or fasting glucose. The increases in microalbuminuria were continuous throughout the range of postchallenge blood glucose (25).

TREATMENT

Morbidly obese children, especially those with evidence of the metabolic syndrome, may be at particular risk for progression of renal pathology.

Studies in adult diabetic patients have shown that treatment of hypertension decreases the amount of protein excretion and slows the rate of renal impairment (16). Microalbuminuria correlates with blood pressure in adults, and reduction in microalbuminuria is achieved via use of antihypertensive drugs (20).

There are no specific guidelines for obese children with microalbuminuria. The American Academy of Pediatrics (AAP) guidelines for Native American children with type 2 diabetes recommend the following (26):

> After confirmation of microalbuminuria by elevated microalbumin/creatinine ratio on two studies and ruling out other primary renal causes of microalbuminuria, consideration of treatment with ACE inhibitors is recommended, bearing in mind that ACE inhibitors are teratogenic. Low dose is recommended to start, with repeat testing to confirm reduction of microalbuminuria and titrate dose. Control of hyperglycemia, hypertension, and smoking cessation are recommended (26).

CASE

Initial Presentation

CB is a 17-year-old African American young woman who is new to your practice. On her first visit, you note her marked obesity and increased difficulty maneuvering around the office. Her weight is 275 lb (>95th percentile) and height is 5 ft 1 in (10th percentile), giving her a BMI of 52.0 (>99th percentile). She is mildly hypertensive, with a blood pressure of 128/82 mm Hg [>95th percentile (126/84 mm Hg) systolic and >90th percentile (122/79 mm Hg) diastolic]. She and her mother note that CB has been "large since birth" and that there are many large relatives in the family. CB is a senior in high school and hopes to graduate and pursue cosmetology as a career. She skips breakfast, and often skips lunch, and then usually eats fast food after school and may or may not eat dinner with the family. Her main beverage during the day is regular soda. The family history is positive for morbid obesity and type 2 diabetes; in fact, her mother is taking insulin, and two of her grandparents passed away from diabetes-related cardiovascular disease.

Review of systems indicates sleep disturbance with snoring, orthopnea, and daytime somnolence; her periods are irregular; and she has noted an increase in fatigue over the past several months, which has prompted this visit to your office. On physical examination, you find that she has acanthosis nigricans of her neck and axilla and marked central obesity. You perform a random glucose by fingerstick in the office and it is 155 mg/dL. You order a 2-hour glucose tolerance test, a lipid panel, and spot urine for creatinine and albumin, along with liver function studies and an a.m. cortisol, blood urea nitrogen (BUN), and creatinine and androgens.

You tell CB she is at increased risk for diabetes and has elevated blood pressure; you explain the etiology and describe the laboratory studies you are ordering. You ask her what these findings mean to her, and CB says she is scared because she has seen what happened to her grandparents. You describe several options to start: lifestyle management, including eliminating soda and sugared beverages, decreasing the intake of fast food, and eating regular meals. She and her mother decide to eliminate soda by buying only diet drinks for the house. You ask her to have her laboratory tests done as soon as possible and schedule an appointment for 2 weeks. You also schedule a sleep study to evaluate her possible sleep apnea and make an appointment with the nutritionist.

Second Visit

CB returns in 2 weeks. Her weight is down about 2 lb, placing her at 273 lb. Her blood pressure is 127/85 mm Hg (>95th percentile systolic and diastolic pressure). Her test results have come back, showing that she has impaired glucose tolerance and insulin resistance with a 2-hour glucose of 164 mg/dL and elevated insulin. Her spot urine shows microalbuminuria, and the rest of her laboratory values are within normal limits.

She has stopped all but a few sodas and occasional juices. She also met with the nutritionist and has begun to keep diet records and decrease her fast food consumption, noting that they talked about her blood pressure and decreasing sodium in her diet.

Her blood pressure is still elevated and she has microalbuminuria. You start treatment with an ACE inhibitor, carefully explaining that this drug is contraindicated in pregnancy. She denies sexual activity, and you ask her to let you know immediately if this changes so you can stop the medicine. CB and her mother express interest in seeing the nutritionist again; you have them schedule this appointment and another appointment with you in 2 weeks.

Third Visit

CB and her mother return, and CB's weight is down another pound. She is taking her antihypertensive medication and following a lower sodium diet. Her blood pressure is 123/79 mm Hg. She has scheduled the sleep study for the following week and, right before your visit with her, has met with the nutritionist, who gave her some meal plans and ideas for breakfast and lunch at school.

You begin to talk about exercise, and she asks what she should do. You suggest adding some walking to her after-school routine, and she is interested. You also talk about screen time and explore other activities she could engage in if she is not watching television. She is unsure but thinks she could call a friend, visit her aunt who lives in the neighborhood, or occasionally go to a friend's house. You schedule an appointment for 1 month and ask her to call you if she is having any shortness of breath or joint problems as she starts to increase her walking. You suggest she begin by walking several minutes per day and increase by 1 minute per day as a way of incorporating the walking into her schedule.

Fourth Visit

CB and her mother check in. She has lost 3 more pounds and is taking her ACE inhibitor; her blood pressure is 120/76 mm Hg. Her sleep study was positive for apnea, and she has been started on bilevel airway pressure (BiPAP). She has begun and continued walking and is feeling more energetic and is not napping regularly after school, as she did in the past. You congratulate her on taking charge of her health and ask what help she needs in "keeping on the right track." She says her mother is helping her with food selection and she would like to come to your office every week to "weigh in." You arrange this with your nurse and plan for CB to return in 2 months for a blood pressure check and follow-up with you. You give her a prescription for spot urine for creatinine and albumin to see if the medication and changes she has made have decreased her microalbuminuria.

REFERENCES

1. Fox CS, Larson MG, Leip EP, Culleton B, Wilson PW, Levy D. Predictors of new-onset kidney disease in a community based population. *JAMA*. 2004;291(7):844–850.
2. Hsu C, McCulloch CE, Iribarren C, Darbinian J, Go AS. Body mass index and risk for end-stage renal disease. *Ann Intern Med*. 2006;144(1):21–28.
3. Amin R, Turner C, van Aken S, Bahu TK, Watts A, Lindsell DR, Dalton RN, Dunger DB. The relationship between microalbuminuria and glomerular filtration rate in young type 1 diabetic subjects: The Oxford Regional Prospective Study. *Kidney Int*. 2005;68(4):1740–1749.
4. Pedrinelli R, Dell'Omo G, Penno G, Mariani M. Nondiabetic microalbuminuria, endothelial dysfunction and cardiovascular disease. *Vasc Med*. 2001;6(4):257–264.
5. Mattock MB, Barnes DJ, Viberti G, Keen H, Burt D, Hughes JM, Fitzgerald AP, Sandhu B, Jackson PG. Microalbuminuria and coronary heart disease in NIDDM: an incidence study. *Diabetes*. 1998; 47(11):1786–1792.
6. Kambham N, Markowitz GS, Valeri AM, Lin J, D'Agati VD. Obesity-related glomerulopathy: an emerging epidemic. *Kidney Int*. 2001;59(4):1498–1509.
7. Adelman RD, Restaino IG, Alon US, Blowey DL. Proteinuria and focal segmental glomerulosclerosis in severely obese adolescents. *J Pediatr*. 2001;138(4):481–485.
8. Ribstein J, duCailar G, Mimran A. Combined renal effects of overweight and hypertension. *Hypertension*. 1995;26(4):610–615.
9. O'Donnell MP, Kasiske BL, Clary MP, Keane WF. Effects of genetic obesity on renal structure and function in Zucker rat II: micropuncture studies. *J Lab Clin Med*. 1985;106(5):605–610.
10. Blanco S, Vaquero M, Gomez-Guerrero C, Lopez D, Egido J, Romero R. Potential role of angiotensin-converting enzyme inhibitors and statins on early podocyte damage in a model of type 2 diabetes mellitus, obesity and mild hypertension. *Am J Hypertens*. 2005;18(4 Pt 1):557–565.

11. Csernus K, Lanyi E, Erhardt E, Molnar D. Effect of childhood obesity and obesity-related cardiovascular risk factors on glomerular and tubular protein excretion. *Eur J Pediatr.* 2005;164(1):44–49.

12. Filler G, Payne RP, Orrbine E, Clifford T, Drukker A, McLaine PN. Changing trends in the referral patterns of pediatric nephrology patients. *Pediatr Nephrol.* 2005;20(5):603–608.

13. de Jong PE, Verhave JC, Pinto-Sietsma SJ, Hillege HL; PREVEND study group. Obesity and target organ damage: the kidney. *Int J Obes Relat Metab Disord.* 2002;26(Suppl 4):S21–24.

14. Adelman RD. Obesity and renal disease. *Curr Opin Nephrol Hypertens.* 2002;11(3):331–335.

15. Wolf G, Chen S, Han DC, Ziyadeh FN. Leptin and renal disease. *Am J Kidney Dis.* 2002;39(1):1–11.

16. Humphrey LL, Ballard DJ. Renal complications in noninsulin dependent diabetes mellitus. *Clin Geriatr Med.* 1990;6(4):807–825.

17. Kamenetzky SA, Bennett PH, Dippe SE, Miller M, LeCompte PA. Clinical and histologic study of diabetes nephropathy in the Pima Indians. *Diabetes.* 1974;23(1):61–68.

18. Lane JT. Microalbuminuria as a marker of cardiovascular and renal risk in type 2 diabetes mellitus: a temporal perspective. *Am J Physiol Renal Physiol.* 2004;286(3):F442–450.

19. Assadi FK. Value of urinary excretion of microalbumin in predicting glomerular lesions in children with isolated microscopic hematuria. *Pediatr Nephrol.* 2005;20(8):1131–1135.

20. Verdecchia P, Rebldi GP. Hypertension and microalbuminuria; the new detrimental duo. *Blood Pressure.* 2004;13(4):198–211.

21. Ritz E. Nephropathy in type 2 diabetes. *J Intern Med.* 1999;245(2):111–126.

22. Hasslacher C, Ritz E, Wahl P, Michael C. Similar risks of nephropathy in patients with type 1 or type 2 diabetes mellitus. *Nephrol Dial Transplant.* 1989;4(10):859–863.

23. Haffner SM, Gonzales C, Valdez RA, Mykkanen L, Hazuda G, Mitchell BD, Monterrosa A, Stern MP. Is microalbuminuria part of the prediabetic state/The Mexico City Diabetes Study. *Diabetologia.* 1993;36(10):1002–1006.

24. Gerstein HC, Mann JF, Yi Q, Zinman B, Dinneen SF, Hoogwerf B, Halle JP, Young J, Rashkow A, Joyce C, Nawaz S, Yusuf S; HOPE Study Investigators. Albuminuria and risk of cardiovascular event, death and heart failure in diabetic and non-diabetic individuals. *JAMA.* 2001;286(4):421–426.

25. Burgert TS, Dziura J, Yeckel C, Taksali SE, Weiss R, Tamborlane W, Caprio S. Microalbuminuria in pediatric obesity: prevalence and relation of other cardiovascular risk factors. *Int J Obes.* 2006; 30(2):273–280.

26. Gahagan S, Silverstein J. Prevention and treatment of type 2 diabetes mellitus in children, with special emphasis on American Indian and Alaska Native children. American Academy of Pediatrics Committee on Native American Child Health. *Pediatrics.* 2003;112(4):e328–e347.

12

Neurologic Complications

The central nervous system is the control center for energy regulation. Initially, case studies suggested the association between hypothalamic injury or tumor and obesity (1). Animal studies confirmed this association with specific lesions in the hypothalamic nuclei, producing unique hypothalamic obesity syndromes (2). The discovery of leptin (3) confirmed the pivotal role of the hypothalamus in energy regulation. The hypothalamus serves as a central relay receiving input from peripheral energy stores and cerebral cortex, regulating feeding behavior, insulin secretion, and autonomic and sympathetic activity.

> Damage to the hypothalamus and central nervous system can disrupt this finely tuned system and result in obesity.

HYPOTHALAMIC OBESITY

State of the Problem

In animal studies, rats that undergo bilateral lesions of the ventromedial hypothalamus (VMH) develop a syndrome of hyperphagia, hyperinsulinemia, and weight gain called "hypothalamic obesity." Obesity due to hypothalamic injury is often associated with other hypothalamic endocrinopathies and is characterized by insulin hypersecretion (4). In a study of children who underwent treatment for primary brain tumors, intermediate- and high-dose radiation to the hypothalamus was a significant factor in body mass index (BMI) increase (4). Rate of BMI increase was not associated with extent of surgery, ventriculoperitoneal shunting, long-term steroid treatment, or chemotherapy. Patients with associated endocrinopathies had greater increases in BMI than those who did not (4).

Etiology

There are at least two distinct hypothalamic syndromes whose manifestations differ depending on which hypothalamic nuclei are affected. Injury to the paraventricular nucleus causes hyperphagia, which is the primary cause of obesity, and when overeating is prevented, obesity does not develop (2).

Injury to the ventral medial nucleus (VMN), in contrast, causes increased activity of the vagal efferent system with greater insulin secretion and reduced thermogenesis. The ventral medial nucleus is also the site of growth hormone–releasing hormone (GHRH) release, and destruction of this nucleus is also associated with decreased growth hormone secretion (2). If lesions are large enough, additional endocrine abnormalities can be seen, including disruption of reproductive function and adrenal and thyroid dysfunction.

In the 1940s, lesions in the VMH were identified as leading to obesity (5). VMH lesions can affect adipocyte function. In rats, VMH lesions resulted in a biphasic response. In the initial stages, insulin level, insulin receptor number, and insulin-stimulated glucose transport and glucose oxidation were increased, contributing to greater lipogenesis. Thereafter, insulin binding and glucose transport decreased to control levels, but insulin-stimulated glucose oxidation remained reduced (6). Decreased glucose tolerance after VMH lesions has been reported in animals and humans (1,7). Hypothalamic lesions of the VMH in mice resulted in marked increases in ob gene product (leptin) secretion (8). Leptin, ghrelin, and insulin affect neuropeptide Y in the arcuate nucleus, allowing signal transduction from peripheral afferent energy signals to affect efferent sympathetic and vagal nerve modulation of appetite and energy balance (9). The exact mechanism of this is unclear; it is thought that increased vagal tone with stimulation of beta cells and hyperinsulinemia may be the cause of weight gain (10). Bilateral vagotomy can reverse obesity in this case (11).

Leptin may be involved in the hyperphagia seen in children with suprasellar injury. Significantly elevated levels of leptin relative to BMI were found in a study of children with suprasellar injury in contrast to those with intrasellar injury and controls. It was hypothesized that a decrease in hypothalamic leptin receptors due to injury resulted in increased neuropeptide Y and reduced corticotropin-releasing hormone, causing hyperphagia (12). In contrast, in a study of obese children with and without hypothalamic obesity, no difference was found between fasting total ghrelin levels, fasting insulin levels, or leptin levels (13). There is some evidence that animals with hypothalamic obesity have a reduction in spontaneous activity (14) as well as lowered rates of lipolysis when exercised (15).

Definition

- **Hypothalamic obesity**—Obesity developing as a result of a pathologic process or treatment involving the hypothalamus.

Clinical Manifestations

Hypothalamic obesity has been defined as obesity resulting from an injury to the hypothalamus by tumor, surgery, or radiation. Symptoms that have been reported in patients with hypothalamic obesity due to tumors include the following (16):

• Headache
• Impaired vision
• Impaired reproductive function
• Diabetes insipidus
• Somnolence
• Behavioral change
• Impaired growth
• Convulsions

Hypothalamic obesity has been associated with trauma (16). Inflammatory diseases such as sarcoidosis, tuberculosis, arachnoiditis, and encephalitis have also been linked to the development of hypothalamic obesity (16).

Solid tumors involving the hypothalamus are causes of hypothalamic obesity as well, with craniopharyngioma being the most common (16). Craniopharyngiomas arise from cells that lie between the pars anterior and the pars distalis and are composed of the remnants of Rathke's pouch. The frequency of obesity associated with craniopharyngioma has been reported from 0% to 40% (16). Children with brain tumors are at high risk for development of obesity after treatment (17). Risk factors include type of tumor (craniopharyngioma), hypothalamic location, extent of surgery, hypothalamic irradiation exceeding 51 Gy, and presence of hypothalamic endocrinopathies. Young age at diagnosis is also a risk factor (17).

Obesity is also a "late effect" in children with cancer.

Up to 47% of young adults with childhood acute lymphoblastic leukemia (ALL) had, at their final height, BMI measurements exceeding the 85th percentile (18). Overweight or obesity as a late effect of ALL has been linked to cranial irradiation (4); it may be increased in those survivors considered growth hormone deficient (18).

A paraneoplastic syndrome involving hypothalamic dysfunction associated with neuroblastoma has been reported (19). Paraneoplastic neurologic disorders develop in association with a neoplasm without direct invasion by tumor and are believed to be autoimmune disorders. Idiopathic hypothalamic dysfunctions linked with neural crest tumors include obesity, central hypoventilation, hypersomnia, hyperphagia, behavior change, abnormal thermoregulation, decreased sensitivity to pain, and hypernatremia. Other manifestations have included hyperprolactinemia, seizures, scoliosis, precocious puberty, and growth hormone deficiency (19).

Treatment

Weight gain after hypothalamic injury can be rapid and hard to control (20,21). In a study of children who had sustained central nervous system injury as a result of tumor, surgery, or irradiation and had evidence of hypothalamic injury, an average weight gain of 6 kg per 6 months was noted (10). When children were treated with octreotide, a long-acting somatostatin analog that attenuates insulin release, the average weight loss was 4.8 kg per 6 months (10). In one series of children treated for craniopharyngioma, 53% were obese and 23% were overweight, and both these groups had greater abdominal obesity and dyslipidemia [higher triglycerides, lower high-density lipoprotein (HDL)] than controls (22). Hyperphagia is not unusual in this population after surgery, despite pituitary hormone replacement (23).

IMPACT ON WEIGHT MANAGEMENT

Development of severe obesity affects both quality of life and long-term morbidity in these patients (24). Strategies for diet, exercise, and close follow-up for obesity are warranted.

Case

Initial Presentation

DS is a 10-year-old African American boy who has recently undergone treatment for craniopharyngioma. He comes to your office for follow-up and for a school physical. His current weight is 150 lb (>95th percentile) and his height is 5 ft (95th percentile); the BMI is 29.3 (>95th percentile). His blood pressure is 119/68 mm Hg. He is taking desmopressin (DDAVP) and thyroid medication prescribed by the endocrinologist. He is excited about returning to school and wants to play basketball this coming season.

Review of systems reveals that he is snoring, with some daytime somnolence and napping after school; his mother is not sure if he has apnea. His mother notes that before his diagnosis, he was normal weight and very active; she notes that he "can't stay away from food" and seems to always want larger portions and second helpings. You see that he has gained 40 lb in the 6 months since his surgery. The family history is positive for diabetes in two grandparents and hypertension in aunts and uncles. On physical examination, DS is a cheerful young man but does become somewhat sad when he talks about how his stamina for physical activity has decreased. He has normal findings on physical examination except for increased central obesity and scars from his craniotomy. He has not yet entered puberty.

You review his diet and activity history and note that his predominant beverage is regular soda. He has no outdoor time and is having about 6 to 8 hours of screen time (mostly television) per day. His mother is concerned about the health effects of his obesity added to the major effects of his tumor, which have resulted in difficulties with learning and memory. DS is mostly concerned about his ability to play sports.

After going over causes of obesity, including his increased risk from his tumor and treatment as well as from his family history, you present some possible changes. DS and his mother think they could eliminate the soda, changing to diet soda because DS does not like to drink water. Planning to see DS again in 1 month, you start with this change and request laboratory test results from his most recent endocrine appointment. You also have his mother call to schedule a sleep study for DS.

One Month Later

One month later DS comes to your office reporting that he has cut back to almost no regular sodas. He has gained 3 lb. His physical examination is essentially unchanged except for a 2-in. decrease in his waist measurement. He is disappointed, but you emphasize that this rate of weight gain is half of what he had been gaining. You have reviewed his laboratory studies, which show that he has elevated insulin but normal glucose, indicating insulin resistance; he also has a triglyceride level of 212 mg/dL, with a normal cholesterol and slightly decreased HDL of 33 mg/dL. His liver enzymes are normal. He had his sleep study the week before; the study revealed that he has sleep apnea, and you review the results with DS and his mother and arrange an appointment to initiate bilevel airway pressure (BiPAP). You praise him for the changes he has made, and the three of you discuss decreasing portion sizes and substituting lower calorie snacks for those he has been eating. Television watching is a major trigger for DS's eating, and you ask him to try limiting his television time. DS gets upset and feels he cannot reduce his television watching at all. You then explore other activities DS might enjoy, such as going to the YMCA or Boys and Girls Club; he responds more positively, and his mother agrees to look into these activities. You schedule the next visit in 1 month and ask the mother to call if any problems or difficulties arise.

Follow-up Visits

About 2 weeks later, you get a call from DS's mother; she says that DS has been complaining of right knee pain and she has noticed him limping once or twice. You ask her to come to the office right away. When DS comes in, you see that he is limping; you send him immediately for x-ray studies, which come back positive for slipped capital femoral epiphysis (SCFE). DS and his mother go right to the hospital, and he is admitted for pinning of his right hip.

You see DS 1 month after surgery, and he is in the process of following up with his physical therapy (PT). His weight is up 4 lb, and he is discouraged both because of the weight and the current limitations to physical activity. He agrees to come to your office weekly for a weight check after his PT appointment, and you schedule an appointment for him with a nutritionist. DS seems somewhat depressed; you ask about this, and he admits he has been feeling pretty sad; there is no suicidal ideation. You ask if he would like to talk about his situation and feelings with a counselor and he agrees, so you schedule an appointment.

You continue to follow up DS monthly as you help him and his family work through his medical issues and continue to focus on family-based lifestyle change for his weight.

PSEUDOTUMOR CEREBRI

State of the Problem

Pseudotumor cerebri can be a complication of obesity that, if untreated, can result in visual impairment or blindness. In a survey of the general population in Louisiana and Iowa in the 1980s, the incidence of pseudotumor was 0.9 per 100,000 people. The prevalence rose to 19 per 100,000 in the population of adult women who were 20% or more over their ideal body weight (25). A Canadian study estimated the incidence of pseudotumor in children by age and gender. In boys age 2 to 11, the incidence was 0.4 per 100,000 child-years of exposure; in girls age 2 to 11, it was 1.1. Girls also had a higher estimated incidence than boys in the adolescent period, with the incidence in girls being 2.2 per 100,000 child-years of exposure and in boys being 0.8. (26).

Definition

- **Pseudotumor cerebri**—Idiopathic increased intracranial pressure associated with papilledema, a normal cerebrospinal fluid (CSF), and the absence of ventricular enlargement (Fig. 12.1).

Etiology

Several mechanisms have been proposed for the increased incidence of pseudotumor cerebri in obese patients. In a group of female patients undergoing bariatric surgery for pseudotumor cerebri, intracranial pressure, urinary bladder pressure,

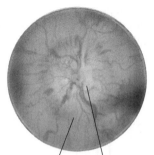

Clear focus here   Clear focus here
at −1 diopter   at + 3 diopters

+ 3 − (−1) = 4, therefore, a
disc elevation of 4 diopters

FIG. 12.1. Papilledema. (From Bickley LS, Szilagyi PG. Bates' *guide to physical examination and history taking,* 8th ed. Philadelphia: Lippincott Williams & Wilkins; 2002.)

transesophageal and pleural pressures, and central venous and pulmonary artery pressures were all elevated compared with normal values and control patients. This supports a hypothesis that obese patients with pseudotumor cerebri have increased intra-abdominal pressure, which may lead to higher pleural and cardiac filling pressures, impeding venous return from the brain, which may cause intracranial venous pressure elevations leading to pseudotumor cerebri (27).

Papilledema has been associated with obstructive sleep apnea. The mechanism is thought to be episodic nocturnal hypoxemia and hypercarbia causing cerebral vasodilatation that results in increased intracranial pressure (28). In a group of obese women with intracranial hypertension, inflammatory markers and opening CSF pressure were increased and the subarachnoidal space was decreased on magnetic resonance imaging (MRI) when compared with control patients (29).

In adult women, polycystic ovarian syndrome (PCOS) and coagulation disorders, often augmented by exogenous estrogens or pregnancy, are associated with pseudotumor cerebri (30).

Clinical Presentation

Pseudotumor cerebri is a diagnosis of exclusion. Other causes of increased intracranial hypertension must be ruled out before this diagnosis can be made (Table 12.1) (31–34).

Lumbar puncture should be performed only after ensuring that there is no intracranial lesion or mass. The diagnosis of pseudotumor is defined by the modified Dandy criteria (Table 12.2) (35).

Patients with pseudotumor cerebri may present with headache, vomiting, blurred vision, and/or diplopia. Loss of peripheral visual fields and reduction in visual acuity may be present (36). Transient obscuration of vision (TOV) may occur and is described as transient blurring or complete loss of vision in one or both eyes for a few seconds, often occurring when the patient bends over or rolls the eyes (37). Patients may also see spots, shadows, or other disturbances in their field of vision (38). Cranial nerve deficits may also be present at presentation and can include bilateral or unilateral sixth nerve palsy, acute esotropia with full abduction, skew deviation, and seventh cranial nerve palsy (39).

TABLE 12.1. *Causes of increased intracranial hypertension*

Idiopathic pseudotumor cerebri	Gliomatosis cerebri (32)
Neurologic disease	Anaplastic oligodendroglioma (33)
Dural venous sinus thrombosis due to otitis media, mastoiditis, head trauma	Glioblastoma multiforme (34)
	Malnutrition
Meningitis	Systemic lupus erythematosis
Arteriovenous malformation	Addison's disease
Diffuse neoplastic process	Severe anemia (aplastic or iron deficiency)
	Occult pseudotumor cerebri (no papilledema)

Reprinted with permission from Distelmaier F, Sengler U, Messing-Juenger M, et al. Pseudotumor cerebri as an important differential diagnosis of papilledema in children. *Brain Dev.* 2006;29:190–195.

TABLE 12.2. *Modified Dandy criteria*

A. Signs and symptoms of increased intracranial pressure
B. Absence of localized findings on neurologic examination
C. Absence of deformity, displacement, or obstruction of the ventricular system in otherwise normal neurodiagnostic studies (MRI) (33), except for increased CSF pressure (normal CSF composition without evidence of infection, inflammation or malignancy)
D. Alert and oriented patient; no other cause of increased intracranial pressure present

MRI, magnetic resonance imaging; CSF, cerebrospinal fluid.
Reprinted with permission from Baker RS, Carter D, Hendricks EB, Buncic JR. Visual loss in pseudotumor cerebri of childhood. A follow up study. *Arch Ophthalmol.* 1985;103:1681–1686.

In some cases, neck, shoulder, and back pain has also been reported (40). Although papilledema is part of the pathologic picture, it may not occur on presentation with the other symptoms.

Obesity has been reported in 29.6% of children with pseudotumor cerebri (41). In a case-controlled series of adolescents and adults, obesity and recent weight gain were the only factors found significantly more often in patients than in controls (42).

Various drugs have been associated with increased risk for pseudotumor cerebri (Table 12.3) (37,43,44), including growth hormone, nalidixic acid, ciprofloxacin, and tetracycline. Steroid withdrawal after long-term administration has also been reported as a cause (37,39), as well as vitamin A and isotretinoin therapy (45,46). Some patients experience a prolonged course of headache and visual disturbance and may have permanent visual defects (47).

Primary headaches may be more common in the obese population. Obese adults in a bariatric surgical series had a higher incidence of migraine and tension headaches when compared with normal weight controls. Migraine is the predominant headache, with a high incidence of headaches that were considered incapacitating (48). In a population study, BMI was associated with frequency but not incidence of migraine headaches, with a fivefold increase in headaches in the obese versus the normal weight group. Severity also increased, with doubling of pain in the morbidly obese compared with normal weight adults as well as increases in photophobia and phonophobia (49).

TABLE 12.3. *Medications associated with the development of pseudotumor cerebri*

Vitamin A	Lithium
Isoretinoin	Levothyroxine
All-*trans*-retinoic acid	Leuproelin
Tetracycline	Growth hormone
Minocycline	Corticosteroids
Doxycycline	Levonorgestrel implant
Ciprofloxacin	Danocrine (27,44)
Sulfa antibacterials	Thyroxin (27,44)
Nalidixic acid	

Reprinted with permission from Friedman DI. Medication-induced intracranial hypertension in dermatology. *Am J Clin Dermatol.* 2005;6:29–37.

Treatment

Treatment of pseudotumor cerebri is with acetazolamide (50), and weight loss leads to remission of symptoms (51). In severe cases, a lumboperitoneal shunt may be needed until pharmacologic treatment and weight loss become effective. Weight loss will correct pseudotumor cerebri, and in some cases pseudotumor cerebri has been an indication for bariatric surgery (52).

Lumboperitoneal shunting may be needed to treat pseudotumor cerebri if medical management is not effective and intracranial pressure remains elevated (53,54).

Optic nerve sheath fenestration is a treatment used to relieve papilledema and optic nerve damage. It has been shown to stabilize or improve vision in adults, especially those with chronic disc edema and severe or progressive vision loss (55).

Case

Initial Presentation

LT is a 16-year-old sophomore in high school who comes to your office for a football physical. LT's weight is 275 lb and he is 5 ft 8 in. tall. His BMI is 41.8; his blood pressure is 122/76 mm Hg. His mother is with him and says he has gained about 30 lb this past year and the football coach is planning to start him on the varsity defense. LT has no allergies and is not taking any medication. LT's family history is positive for gallbladder disease in a maternal grandmother and hypertension in the paternal grandfather, and the mother notes that the father's whole family is "big," with several aunts and uncles weighing more than 350 lb. She and LT are not at all concerned about his size.

On review of systems, LT notes that he has "some headaches;" he snores at night and sleeps on two or three pillows. You begin the physical examination and immediately note that LT has bilateral papilledema. There are no localizing neurologic signs. The rest of the physical examination yields findings within normal limits except for his obesity. You perform a visual field check by confrontation, and it seems that there may be some peripheral field loss of vision.

You have your staff call the neurologist at the hospital, who agrees to see LT right away. You explain the papilledema to LT and his mother, emphasizing that you are very concerned about the findings.

LT goes to the neurologist, who orders an MRI. You check in with LT's mother, who says the MRI is normal and the neurologist is going to perform a spinal tap; you reassure her that this is an important diagnostic test. Later that afternoon, you make rounds at the hospital and check in with LT and the neurologist, who reports that LT has pseudotumor cerebri and has been started on acetazolamide (Diamox). You arrange to see LT in your office in about 1 week.

A week later, LT and his mother return to your office. His headaches have disappeared; he is still taking acetazolamide. You begin by discussing pseudotumor cerebri and the relationship to his weight; you also express concern about possible sleep apnea from his initial history. LT and his mother are worried; they agree to a sleep study and want to address his weight gain. You arrange for a sleep study and go over LT's diet and activity. It turns out that LT routinely skips breakfast, eats a school lunch and buys extra chips and two juices, and usually stops at the corner store after school for a snack. His snack consists of a soda and hot dog, and he eats dinner with his family, usually taking two helpings. He snacks at night while on the computer, usually leftovers, and drinks one to two regular sodas before going to bed. You go over several options for working on lowering his weight; these include changing from regular to diet soda, substituting lower calorie food for snacks, and beginning to eat breakfast. LT and his mother say that they can choose different snack food, but the soda will be a challenge. You ask if they have ever tried diet soda, and LT says he has not. You ask him to try some varieties of diet drinks and see what he thinks. You give LT and mom a list of low-calorie snack food to have in the house and some ideas for breakfast. You arrange to see LT in 1 month.

One Month Later

One month later, LT returns. His weight is down 4 lb and he has had his sleep study, which was positive for sleep apnea. You arrange to start him on bilevel airway pressure (BiPAP) and ask him how he lost weight. LT says he has been drinking only one regular soda per day and has "lightened up" on his snacks. Mom has also been reducing the amount of food she cooks for dinner, so there is less for second helpings and no leftovers. He has seen the neurologist, is no longer taking acetazolamide, and is not having any headaches. You encourage him to think about joining a conditioning program at the YMCA and arrange to see him again in 1 month.

Follow-up Visits

One month later, LT has lost another 4 lb. He has been working out at the YMCA and enjoying it. He is not as hungry as before and is happier with a single portion at dinner. He is, however, having trouble wearing his BiPAP, although he can notice the improvement in his energy level when he does. You discuss his bedtime routine and suggest some relaxation techniques to see if this will help the BiPAP use. You schedule a follow-up visit for 1 month.

The visit 1 month later starts with LT telling you that he is wearing his BiPAP at night and feels better. His mother notes that he is less irritable and seems to be doing better in school. He is going to the YMCA three or four times per week and has begun a weight-training program there. His weight is down another 5 lb. You arrange a 6-week follow-up.

REFERENCES

1. Bray GA, Gallagher TF. Manifestations of hypothalamic obesity in man: a comprehensive investigation of eight patients and a review of the literature. *Medicine (Baltimore).* 1975;54(4):301–330.
2. Bray GA. Genetic hypothalamic and endocrine features of clinical and experimental obesity. In: Swaab DF, Hofman M, Mirmiran R, Leewen RR, eds. *Progress in Brain Research,* Vol. 93. Amsterdam: Elsevier; 1992:333–340.

3. Zhang Y, Porenca R, Maffei M, Barone M, Leopold L, Friedman JM. Positional cloning of the mouse obese gene and its human homologue. *Nature.* 1994;372(6505):425–432. Erratum in *Nature.* 374:479.
4. Lustig RH, Post SR, Sirvannaboom K, Rose SR, Danish RK, Burghen GA, Xiong X, Wu S, Merchantt TE. Risk factors for the development of obesity in children surviving brain tumors. *J Clin Endocrinol Metab.* 2003;88(2):611–616.
5. Hetherington AW, Ranson SW. Hypothalamic lesions and adiposity in the rat. *Anat Rec.* 1940;78: 149–172.
6. Kasuga M, Inoue S, Akanuma Y, Kosaka K. Insulin receptor function and insulin effects on glucose metabolism in adipocytes from ventromedial hypothalamus lesioned rats. *Endocrinology.* 1980; 107(5):1549–1555.
7. Komorowski JM. Blood sugar and immunoreactive insulin in women with hypothalamic, maternal and simple obesity Part I. *Endokrinologie.* 1977;70(2):182–191.
8. Maffei M, Fei H, Lee GH, Dani C, Leroy P, Zhang Y, Proenca R, Negrel R, Ailhaud G, Friedman JM. Increased expression in adipocytes of ob RNA in mice with lesions of the hypothalamus and with mutation at the db locus. *Proc Natl Acad Sci U S A.* 1995;92(15):6957–6960.
9. Menyhert J, Wittmann G, Hrabovszky E, Keller E, Liposits Z, Fekete C. Interconnection between orexigenic neuropeptide Y and anorexigenic alpha-melanocyte stimulating hormone synthesizing neuronal systems of the human hypothalamus. *Brain Res.* 2006;1076(1):101–105.
10. Lustig RH, Rose SR, Burghen GA, Velasquez-Mieyer P, Broome DC, Smith K, Li H, Hudson MM, Heideman RI, Kun LE. Hypothalamic obesity in children caused by cranial insult; altered glucose and insulin dynamics and reversal by a somatostatin agonist. *J Pediatr.* 1999;135:162–168.
11. Inoue S, Bray GA. The effects of sub diaphragmatic vagotomy in rats with ventromedial hypothalamic obesity. *Endocrinology.* 1977;100(1):108–114.
12. Roth C, Wilken B, Hanefeld F, Schroter W, Leonhardt U. Hyperphagia in children with craniopharyngioma is associated with hyperleptinaemia and a failure in the down regulation of appetite. *Eur J Endocrinol.* 1998;138(1):89–91.
13. Kanumakala S, Greaves R, Pedreira C, Donath S, Warne GL, Zacharin MR, Harris M. Fasting ghrelin levels are not elevated in children with hypothalamic obesity. *J Clin Endocrinol Metab.* 2005; 90(5):2691–2695.
14. Gladfelter WE. Locomotor response to changes in food intake and ambient temperature in rats with hypothalamic lesions. *Physiol Behav.* 1978;20(3):227–231.
15. Jenkins RR, Lamb DR. Effects of physical training on hypothalamic obesity in rats. *Eur J Appl Physiol.* 1982;48(3):355–359.
16. Bray G. Syndromes of hypothalamic obesity in man. *Pediatr Ann.* 1984;13(7):525–536.
17. Didi M, Didcock E, Davies HA, Oglivy-Stuart AL, Wales JK, Shalet SM. High incidence of obesity in young adults after treatment of acute lymphoblastic leukemia in childhood. *J Pediatr.* 1995;127(1):63–67.
18. Link K, Moell C, Garwicz S, Cavallin-Stahl E, Bjork J, Thilen U, Ahren B, Erfurth EM. Growth hormone deficiency predicts cardiovascular risk in young adults treated for acute lymphoblastic leukemia in childhood. *J Clin Endocrinol Metab.* 2004;89(10):5003–5012.
19. Sirvent N, Berard E, Chastagner P, Feillet F, Wagner K, Sommelet D. Hypothalamic dysfunction associated with neuroblastoma; evidence for a new paraneoplastic syndrome. *Med Pediatr Oncol.* 2003;40(5):326–328.
20. Bray GA, Inoue S, Nishizawa Y. Hypothalamic obesity; the autonomic hypothesis and the lateral hypothalamus. *Diabetologia.* 1981;20(Suppl):366–377.
21. Lustig RH. Obesity in childhood cancer survivors. *Pediatr Endocrinol Rev.* 2006(Suppl 2):306–311.
22. Srinivasan S, Ogle GD, Garnett SP, Briody JN, Lee JW, Cowell CT. Features of the metabolic syndrome after childhood craniopharyngioma. *J Clin Endocrinol Metab.* 2004;89(1):81–86.
23. Muller HL, Bueb K, Bartels U, Roth C, Harz K, Graaf N, Korinthenberg R, Bettendorf M, Kuhl J, Gutjahr P, Sorensen N, Calaminus G. Obesity after childhood craniopharyngioma–German multicenter study on pre-operative risk factors and quality of life. *Klin Padiatr.* 2001;213:244–249.
24. Muller HL, Gebhardt U, Etavard-Gorris N, Korenke E, Warmuth-Metz M, Kolb R, Sorensen N, Calaminus G. Prognosis and sequela in patients with childhood craniopharyngioma—results of HIT_ENDO and update on KRANIOPHARYNGEOM 2000. *Klin Padiatr.* 2004;216(6):343–348.
25. Durcan FJ, Corbett JJ, Wall M. The incidence of pseudotumor cerebri: population studies in Iowa and Louisiana. *Arch Neurol.* 1988;45(8):875–877.
26. Gordon K. Pediatric pseudotumor cerebri: descriptive epidemiology. *Can J Neurol Sci.* 1997;24(3): 219–221.

27. Sugerman HJ, DeMaria EJ, Felton WL, Nakatsuka M, Sismanis A. Increased intra-abdominal pressure and cardiac filling pressures in obesity associated pseudotumor cerebri. *Neurology.* 1997;49(2): 507–511.
28. Purvin VA, Kawasaki A, Yee RD. Papilledema and obstructive sleep apnea syndrome. *Arch Ophthalmol.* 2000;118(12):11626–11630.
29. Hannerz J, Greitz D, Ericson K. Is there a relationship between obesity and intracranial hypertension? *Int J Obes Relat Metab Disord.* 1995;19(4):240–244.
30. Glueck CJ, Iyengar S, Goldenberg N, Smith LS, Wang P. Idiopathic intracranial hypertension's associations with coagulation disorders and polycystic ovary syndrome. *J Lab Clin Med.* 2003;142(1): 35–45.
31. Distelmaier F, Sengler U, Messing-Juenger M, Assmann B, Mayatepek E, Rosenbaum T. Pseudotumor cerebri as an important differential diagnosis of papilledema in children. *Brain Dev.* 2006;29(3): 190–195.
32. Weston P, Lear J. Gliomatosis cerebri or benign intracranial hypertension? *Postgrad Med J.* 1995; 71(836):380–381.
33. Said RR, Rosman NP. A negative cranial computed tomographic scan is not adequate to support a diagnosis of pseudotumor cerebri. *J Child Neurol.* 2004;19(8):609–613.
34. Aroichane M, Miller NR, Eggenberger ER. Glioblastoma multiforme masquerading as pseudotumor cerebri. Case report. *J Clin Neuroophthalmol.* 1993;13(2):105–112.
35. Friedman DI, Jacobson DM. Diagnostic criteria for idiopathic intracranial hypertension. *Neurology.* 2002;59(10):1492–1495.
36. Baker RS, Carter D, Hendricks EB, Buncic JR. Visual loss in pseudotumor cerebri of childhood. A follow up study. *Arch Ophthalmol.* 1985;103(11):1681–1686.
37. Friedman DI. Medication-induced intracranial hypertension in dermatology. *Am J Clin Dermatol.* 2005;6(1):29–37.
38. Handbook of ocular disease management. http://www.revoptom.com/HANDBOOK/SECT53a.HTM (accessed 5/5/06).
39. Bakshi SK, Oak JL, Chawla KP, Kulkarni SD, Apte N. Facial nerve involvement in pseudotumor cerebri. *J Postgrad Med.* 1992;38:144-145.
40. Lessell S. Pediatric pseudotumor cerebri (idiopathic intracranial hypertension). *Surv Ophthalmol.* 1992;37(3):155–166.
41. Scott IU, Siatkowski RM, Eneyni M, Brodsky MC, Lam BL. Idiopathic intracranial hypertension in children and adolescents. *Am J Ophthalmol.* 1997;124(2):253–255.
42. Wall M. Idiopathic intracranial hypertension. *Semin Ophthalmol.* 1995;109:251–259.
43. Hamed LM, Glaser JS, Schatz NJ, Perez TH. Pseudotumor cerebri induced by danazol. *Am J Ophthalmol.* 1989;107(2):105–110.
44. Raghavan S, DiMartino-Nardi J, Saenger P, Linder B. Pseudotumor cerebri in an infant after L-thyroxine therapy for transient neonatal hypothyroidism. *J Pediatr.* 1997;130(3):478–480.
45. Morrice G Jr, Havener WH, Kapetansky F. Vitamin A intoxication as a cause of pseudotumor cerebri. *JAMA.* 1960;173:1802–1805.
46. Roytman M, Frumkin A, Bohn TG. Pseudotumor cerebri caused by isotretinoin. *Cutis.* 1988;42(5): 399–400.
47. Skau M, Brennum J, Gjerris F, Jensen R. What is new about idiopathic intracranial hypertension? An updated review of mechanism and treatment. *Cephalalgia.* 2006;26(4):384–399.
48. Peres MF, Lerario DD, Garrido AB, Zukerman E. Primary headaches in obese patients. *Arq Neuropsiquiatr.* 2005;63(4):931–933.
49. Bigal ME, Libberman JN, Lipton RB. Obesity and migraine a population study. *Neurology.* 2006; 66(4):545–550.
50. Schoeman JF. Childhood pseudotumor cerebri clinical and intracranial pressure response to acetazolamide and furosemide treatment in a case series. *J Child Neurol.* 1994;99:130–134.
51. Johnson LN, Krohel GB, Madsen RW, March GA. The role of weight loss and acetazolamide in the treatment of idiopathic intracranial hypertension (pseudotumor cerebri). *Ophthalmology.* 1998;105: 2313–2317.
52. Bouldin MJ, Ross LA, Sumrall CD, Looustalot FV, Low AK, Land KK. The effect of obesity surgery on obesity comorbidity. *Am J Med Sci.* 2006;331(4):183–193.
53. McGirt MJ, Woodworth G, Thomas G, Miller N, Williams M, Rigamonti D. Cerebrospinal fluid shunt placement for pseudotumor cerebri associated intractable headache; predictors of treatment response and an analysis of long-term outcomes. *J Neurosurg.* 2004;101:627–632.
54. Eggenberger ER, Miller NR, Vitale S. Lumboperitoneal shunts for the treatment of pseudotumor cerebri. *Neurology.* 1996;46:1524–1530.
55. Thuente DD, Buckley EG. Pediatric optic nerve sheath decompression. *Ophthalmology.* 2005;112: 724–727.

13

Mental Health Issues

There is a complex relationship between obesity and psychological morbidity.

Psychological conditions can (a) predict later obesity, (b) be consequences of obesity (c) be associated with obesity, and (d) affect obesity treatment. This is not surprising, considering the intricacies of energy regulation, which depends on the ability to regulate eating behavior, hunger, affective states, and interactions with the nutritional environment as well as maintain a balance between physical activity and inactivity, all factors that are vulnerable when mental and social health is impaired (Fig. 13.1).

PREDICTORS

In childhood, factors such as poverty, social stress, and parental neglect have been found to predict adult body mass index (BMI) (1). These social factors also correlate

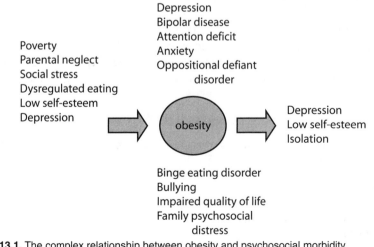

FIG. 13.1. The complex relationship between obesity and psychosocial morbidity.

with child psychopathology. In a longitudinal study, childhood depression was correlated with an increased adult BMI even though there was no difference in childhood BMI between those children who were depressed and nondepressed controls (2). Lissau and Sorensen (2) suggest that parental neglect may cause a psychological state that affects energy balance by either altering behavior that causes overeating and physical inactivity or altering hormonal balance that influences fat storage. It is known that the physiologic reaction to stress is to increase cortisol production, which alters glucose homeostasis, and this may affect eating behavior at the level of the central nervous system in an attempt to reverse stress-induced effects (3).

Depression has clearly been shown to precede the development of obesity.

In a longitudinal study of adolescents in New Zealand, depression in girls in late adolescence conferred a twofold risk of obesity at age 26 years. The risk of adult obesity was also related to the number of episodes of depression these girls experienced. These relationships were not found in boys or in girls in early adolescence (4). In another study of 7th- to 12th-grade adolescents, depressed mood predicted follow-up obesity 1 year later. In contrast, baseline obesity did not predict follow-up depression (5).

Dysregulated eating behavior may also be a risk factor for obesity. In a study of adolescent girls surveyed yearly over 4 years, self-reported dietary restraint, radical weight control behaviors, depressive symptoms, and perceived parental obesity predicated obesity onset. Of interest in this study is that the consumption of high-fat food, binge eating, and exercise frequency were not predictive of later obesity (6). Dysregulated eating may also be a symptom of family stress and/or parental physical or psychological illness.

A negative or low self-concept may predispose children and adolescents to obesity.

In a Canadian population study of adolescents, girls and young adolescents who had a weak self-concept had an increased incidence of depression when studied longitudinally. Low self-concept also predicted physical inactivity among boys and obesity among both boys and girls. Self-esteem was lower among girls than boys (7).

CONSEQUENCES

Obese children and adolescents can develop psychosocial morbidity, which includes the following:

- Depression
- Low self-esteem
- Poor school and social functioning
- Social isolation

In a study of 7th- to 12th-grade adolescents, younger but not older, overweight and obese adolescents ages 12 to 14 had an increased rate of depression, low self-esteem, and poor school and social functioning. Overweight and obese adolescents of all ages had worse self-reported health and functional limitations (8). Overweight adolescents were more likely to be socially isolated than normal weight peers and to have fewer friends. Behaviors not uncommonly seen in obese adolescents, such as increased television viewing and lower sports and club participation, were found to contribute to social isolation in both overweight and normal weight teens (9). One third of obese children and adolescents who sought treatment at an obesity clinic self-reported difficulties with social function and low self-esteem as well as with internalizing symptoms (10).

> Overweight and obesity carry social consequences, which are often linked to psychological morbidity.

Women who had been overweight at ages 16 to 24 in follow-up 7 years later had completed fewer years of school, were less likely to be married, had lower household incomes, and had higher rates of household poverty than the women who had not been overweight, independent of their baseline socioeconomic status and aptitude test scores. Men who had been overweight were less likely to be married (11).

Obesity is also a risk factor for bullying from peers. Associations have been found between BMI and peer victimization, such as withdrawing friendship, spreading rumors or lies, name-calling, teasing, and peer aggression—hitting, kicking or pushing in girls, and verbal bullying in boys. In contrast, obese boys and girls in the older age groups (15 to 16 years) were more likely to perpetrate bullying than normal weight peers (12).

Overall quality of life is often compromised in children and adolescents who are obese.

> The likelihood of having impaired health-related quality of life is 5.5 times greater in obese children and adolescents than in normal weight peers.

Obese children reported lower health-related quality of life scores in all domains—physical, psychosocial, emotional, social, and school functioning—than normal weight children and adolescents. Parents of obese children scored them even lower in these domains (13).

ASSOCIATIONS

Children diagnosed with depression, bipolar disease, and anxiety disorders may be at increased risk for developing obesity. (14). A review of the literature to determine the association of mood disorders and obesity found that children and adolescents with major depression are at risk for developing overweight. Patients with bipolar disease may have higher than average rates of overweight, obesity, and abdominal obesity (14).

> In consequence, an increased incidence of psychological comorbidity may be found in children and families who seek treatment for obesity.

In a study from Turkey of children and adolescents in obesity clinic, about 40% of patients were found to have an anxiety disorder. There was no correlation between the degree of obesity in the child or parents and the frequency of psychiatric disorders. When compared with children with type 1 diabetes, obese children had higher internalized and externalized score and poorer social skills (15).

Patterns of obesity are also associated with specific mental health problems and point to the importance of a longitudinal understanding of the weight gain trajectory. In a longitudinal study of children and adolescents in Appalachia, four weight gain trajectories were identified: normal weight following the standard growth curves, obesity developing in childhood that resolved in adolescence, obesity developing in adolescence, and obesity that developed in childhood and continued through adolescence (chronic obesity). These obesity trajectories were associated with the risk of psychological morbidity. Children who were chronically obese, comprising 15% of the study population, had a greater incidence of oppositional defiant disorder in both girls and boys and a significantly greater rate of depression in boys compared with normal weight boys. Interestingly, there was no difference among the children with various obesity trajectories in gender, family structure, parenting style, family history of mental illness, drug abuse, crime, or traumatic events. Both chronic obesity and childhood obesity were associated with having less educated parents and low family income (16).

> Obese children and adolescents are a heterogeneous population with respect to psychological morbidity.

In a study of an obesity clinic population, children who were depressed had a lower self-esteem than children who were not depressed. As depression increased, self-esteem decreased. Depressed children had increased anxiety and had more perceived behavior problems, such as increased frequency of punishment and difficulty in obeying orders, than nondepressed obese patients. Children in the depressed group also had fewer interests in school and thought their physical appearance was not acceptable. Depression in this group of obese patients did not correlate with age, race, sex, Tanner stage, socioeconomic status, or BMI (17).

Specific eating behaviors may be associated with psychological morbidity. Binge eating is not uncommon in patients with obesity. Adolescents in an obesity treatment program with binge eating had higher levels of depression and anxiety than did adolescents with no binge eating symptoms, as well as lower levels of self-esteem and body-esteem (18). In a group of overweight children (6–10 years) who were not in treatment, one third experienced episodes of loss of control over eating. These children weighed more and had greater body fat than children who did not experience loss of control. They were more likely to be depressed and anxious and had increased body dissatisfaction than children without loss of control. Among these children 5.3% met the criteria for binge eating disorder. These episodes were sporadic and contextual and involved usual foods (19).

Attention deficit disorder (ADD) has been identified as an obesity-related comorbidity. In obese adults in a weight treatment program, the prevalence of ADD was 27.4% and increased to 42.6% in patients with a BMI greater than 40 (20).

In a hospital-based obesity treatment program, more than one half (57.7%) of the obese patients suffered from comorbid attention deficit hyperactivity disorder (ADHD), and the authors speculate that "the characteristic difficulty in regulation found in ADHD may be a risk factor for the development of abnormal eating behaviors leading to obesity" and the authors suggested that "obese children should be screened routinely for ADHD" (21).

IMPACT ON THERAPY

Coexisting psychological conditions, such as stress and depression, can affect food choices and may interfere with behavior change toward a healthier diet. Sweet, energy-dense, high-fat foods can improve mood and mitigate some of the effects of stress and in vulnerable individuals can be self-reinforcing choices (22).

Intervention and therapy for obesity focuses on family-based lifestyle intervention, and children and parents who suffer from depression, anxiety, bipolar illness, and ADD have additional obstacles to overcome in implementing treatment. In a study of children and adolescents in an obesity treatment program, 55% of patients withdrew from treatment. They were more likely to be Medicaid recipients, black, older, and self-report greater depressive symptomatology and lower self-concept (23). In adults, mean weight loss in obese patients with ADD was about one half of those who did not have ADD. Obese adult patients with ADD had more clinic visits and longer treatment duration (20).

Family function can affect treatment, and attention should be paid not only to the child's and adolescent's psychosocial difficulties but also to those of the family. In a study of obese children and adolescents, 41% of children's mothers and 56% of adolescents' mothers reported clinically significant psychological distress. The child's and adolescent's reports of psychological difficulties were strongly associated with the mother's level of psychological distress and/or family socioeconomic status (24).

FAMILY FACTORS CAN ALSO BE SOMEWHAT PROTECTIVE

Family connectedness, parental expectations, and moderate levels of parental monitoring seemed to reduce unhealthy behavior and psychosocial distress (25). Psychosocial factors in obese children and families are common and can be predictive, associated, and/or consequences of obesity. It is important to identify both psychosocial risks and resilience in children, adolescents, and their families so that treatment can be instituted and implementation of lifestyle change can be successful.

CASE

Initial Presentation

GR is a 15-year-old African American boy who comes for a "check-up" because his parents are worried about his decreased energy. Two months ago, his parents had taken him to a psychiatrist, and he was diagnosed with depression and was prescribed fluoxetine (Prozac). His mother is overweight and has recently been diagnosed with diabetes; she has begun insulin therapy, and she says this has really upset GR. His weight at this examination is 106.2 kg (>95th percentile) and his height is 174.8 cm (75th percentile), with a BMI of 35.6 (>95th percentile). Blood pressure is 125/70 mm Hg (<90th percentile). His mother and father are both obese, as are his two older brothers, whose BMIs range from 28 to 35. His family history is positive for diabetes in a paternal grandmother as well as in his mother. Hypertension is a problem for all the great aunts and uncles on his father's side of the family, and his maternal grandfather has cardiovascular disease. One of his brothers has been diagnosed with attention deficit disorder; his maternal grandmother has obsessive-compulsive disorder and depression.

You review his diet history and discover that he is skipping breakfast (no time to eat), buying a school lunch, and eating one to two portions of dinner. He is drinking "a lot" of soda and juice between meals and is snacking at night. He is busy with extracurricular activities, which include the school newspaper and yearbook but is not playing any sports and is watching the television or using the computer "all the time" when he is at home. His parents are concerned about his behavior and report that GR frequently argues with them, daydreams, and demands a lot of attention. He seems to be jealous of his brothers, has low self-esteem, and can be very stubborn. His school performance is declining, and he has recently been put on academic probation. When you ask about homework, GR says he is "not doing any."

He has been getting headaches, and his parents have taken him to a neurologist. His headaches are stress headaches, but his parents are wondering if he has visual integration problems. He has asthma and uses an inhaler as needed. Physical examination reveals that he is a Tanner 5 and has abdominal striae. You acknowledge the parents' concerns about GR's behavior and fatigue and raise the issue of his weight. You decide to order laboratory tests, and you work out a time to see the family in 2 weeks to discuss the results and begin working on a plan for GR.

Two Weeks Later

Two weeks later GR and his mother return, and you review his laboratory studies, which show an elevated fasting total cholesterol of 195 mg/dL. His fasting glucose was normal at 86 mg/dL and his insulin was normal at 14 µU/mL. His thyroid studies and liver enzymes were also within normal limits. You discuss the fact that medically GR is at risk for cardiovascular disease and diabetes based on the family history and that his weight has a direct impact on his risk. This worries GR, especially because his mother already has diabetes. His risk for cardiovascular disease is very much on his mother's mind because his maternal grandfather was just diagnosed with heart failure.

You review the multiple factors that may be influencing GR's weight gain, which include a positive family history of obesity. His parents clearly feel that his inactivity is a major factor in his weight gain, and they are concerned about his lack of energy. They do not really see diet as a problem; GR notes that the fluoxetine has helped him feel less hungry and decrease his night-time eating. You note that depression can be associated with weight gain but also discuss that his decline in school performance, trouble finishing homework, and difficulty with concentration may mean that he also has ADD, especially in light of the positive family history. You suggest that ongoing counseling would be helpful. GR's mother agrees to discuss this with his psychiatrist.

You point out that lack of timed meals and snacks and dysregulated eating work against weight loss. Time management becomes an issue as it relates to the balance between homework, inactivity, and activity and the need for a schedule. As you, GR, and his mother begin to discuss structure and planning meal times, menus, and physical activity, his mother says she thinks she has trouble providing structure because she may have ADD herself; you encourage her to explore this diagnosis.

You work with GR and his mother to set the first goal as weight stabilization using family-based change to institute small changes in nutrition, activity, and inactivity and to remove obstacles to behavior change. The family will set standard meal times and GR will try to have three meals and one after school snack daily. GR agrees, as long as he can still order a school lunch. They will also eliminate calorie-containing juice and soda from the home (an additional benefit for the mother, who has diabetes). He will try to work with a study schedule to finish homework and create opportunities for activity and agrees to begin walking 15 minutes daily. Neither he nor his mother could see any way to limit television or computer time.

You are also continuing to address his other medical follow-up by having him keep diet records to track fat intake to monitor his elevated cholesterol. You arrange a follow-up appointment in 1 month.

One Month Later

One month later the family has canceled the appointment because of the death of the maternal grandfather. On the phone, mom reports that GR initially followed his diet changes and walking program, but this was disrupted by the loss of his grandfather and his family's distress. She notes that GR did see his psychiatrist for evaluation of possible ADD; the diagnosis was made, and he was started on Adderall XR and was still taking his fluoxetine.

Two Months Later

GR returns 1 month later. His weight is 100.4 kg, a decrease of 5.8 kg, and his BMI is 33.4, a decrease of 2.2. His waist measurement is down by 2 in. He reports that he has cut back "drastically" on regular soda consumption; he is trying to make better choices when he eats at restaurants and is trying to find a safe place to walk (his mother is concerned about the neighborhood). He reports that his mood is stable and he is still in counseling. You congratulate GR on his progress and ask if he can continue the changes he has made. You also give him some information on increasing the fiber in his diet and encourage him to try to limit his television/computer time by 1 hour per day. You also spend some time discussing his grief at his grandfather's death.

Follow-up Visits

GR misses his next appointment because of the school's concerns about his missed days, but his mother calls and reports that his medications have been changed to methylphenidate (Concerta), dexmethylphenidate (Focalin), and bupropion (Wellbutrin). She reports that school continues to be stressful, but his mood has improved and his interest in school and activities has increased.

Sixteen weeks after his initial visit, GR returns to the office. He has lost a total of 17.8 lb, and his BMI is 32.3, a decrease of 3.3. His cholesterol is now 184 mg/dL. He plans to increase his walking and continue the changes he has made in his eating schedule and food choices.

You have him check in with a nutritionist to continue support for his nutritional decision making and arrange to see him in 2 months.

REFERENCES

1. Lissau I, Sorensen TIA. Parental neglect during childhood and increased risk of obesity in young adulthood. *Lancet.* 1994;343:324–327.
2. Pine DS, Goldstein RB, Wolk S, Wessman MM. The association between childhood depression and adulthood body mass index. *Pediatrics.* 2001;107:1049–1056.
3. Dallman MF, Pecoraro N, Akana SF, La Fleur SE, Gomez F, Houshyar H, Bell ME, Bhatnagar S, Laugero L, Manalo S. Chronic stress and obesity; a new view of "comfort food". *Proc Natl Acad Sci U S A.* 2003;100(20):11696–11701.
4. Richardson LP, Davis R, Poulton R, McCauley E, Moffitt TE, Caspi A, Connell F. A longitudinal evaluation of adolescent depression and adult obesity. *Arch Pediatr Adolesc Med.* 2003;157:739–745.

5. Goodman E, Whitaker RC. A prospective study of the role of depression in the development and persistence of adolescent obesity. *Pediatrics.* 2002;110:497–504.
6. Stice E, Presnell K, Shaw H, Rohde P. Psychological and behavioral risk factors for obesity onset in adolescent girls: a prospective study. *J Consult Clin Psychol.* 2005;73:195–202.
7. Park J. Adolescent self-concept and health into adulthood. *Health Rep.* 2003;14(Suppl):41–52.
8. Swallen KC, Reither EN, Haas SA, Meier AM. Overweight, obesity and health–related quality of life among adolescents: the National Longitudinal Study of Adolescent Health. *Pediatrics.* 2005;115: 340–347.
9. Strauss RS, Pollack HA. Social marginalization of overweight children. *Arch Pediatr Adolesc Med.* 2003;157:746–752.
10. Zeller MN, Saelens BE, Roehrig H, Kirk S, Daniels SR. Psychological adjustment of obese youth presenting for weight management treatment. *Obes Res.* 2004;12:1576–1586.
11. Gortmaker SL, Must A, Perrin JM, Sobol AM, Dietz WH. Social and economic consequences of overweight in adolescence and young adulthood. *N Engl J Med.* 1993;329:1008–1012.
12. Janssen I, Craig WM, Boyce WF, Pickett W. Associations between overweight and obesity with bullying behaviors in school aged children. *Pediatrics.* 2004;113:1187–1194.
13. Schwimmer JB, Burwinkle T, Varni JW. Health-related quality of life of severely obese children and adolescents. *JAMA.* 2003;289(14):1813–1819.
14. McElroy SL, Kotwal R, Malhotra S, Nelson EB, Keck PE, Nemeroff CB. Are mood disorder and obesity related? A review for the mental health professional. *J Clin Psychiatry.* 2004;45:634–651.
15. Erermis S, Cetin N, Tamar M, Bukusoglu N, Akdeniz F, Goksen D. Is obesity a risk factor for psychopathology among adolescents. *Pediatr Int.* 2004;46:296–301.
16. Mustillo S, Worthman C, Erkanli A, Keeler G, Angold A, Costello EJ. Obesity and psychiatric disorder; developmental trajectories. *Pediatrics.* 2003;111:851–859.
17. Sheslow D, Hassink S, Wallace W, DeLancey E. The relationship between self-esteem and depression in obese children. *Ann N Y Acad Sci.* 1993;699:289–291.
18. Isnard P, Michel G, Frelut ML, Vila G, Falissard B, Naja W, Navarro J, Mouren-Simeoni MC. Binge eating and psychopathology in severely obese adolescents. *Int J Eating Disord.* 2003;34:235–243.
19. Morgan CM, Yanovski SZ, Nguyen TT, McDuffie J, Sebring NG, Jorge MR, Keil M, Yanovski JA. Loss of control over eating, adiposity, and psychopathology in overweight children. *Int J Eating Disord.* 2002;31:430–431.
20. Altfas JR. Prevalence of attention deficit/hyperactivity disorder among adults in obesity treatment. *BMC Psychiatry.* 2002;13,2:9.
21. Agranat-Meged AN, Deitcher C, Goldzweig G, Leibenson L, Stein M, Galili-Weisstub E. Childhood obesity and attention deficit/hyperactivity disorders: a newly described comorbidity in obese hospitalized children. *Int J Eating Disord.* 2005;37:357–359.
22. Leigh Gibson E. Emotional influences on food choice; Sensory, physiological and psychological pathways. *Physiol Behav.* 2006;89(1):53–61.
23. Zeller M, Kirk S, Clator R, Khoury P, Grieme J, Santangelo M, Daniels S. Predictors of attrition from a pediatric weight management program. *J Pediatr.* 2004;144:466–470.
24. Zeller MN, Saelens BE, Roehrig H, Kirk S, Daniels SR. Psychological adjustment of obese youth presenting for weight management treatment. *Obes Res.* 2004;12:1576–1586.
25. Mellin AE, Neumark-Sztainer D, Story M, Ireland M, Resnick MD. Unhealthy behaviors and psychosocial difficulties among overweight adolescents: the potential impact of familial factors. *J Adolesc Health.* 2002;31:145–153.

14

Specific Genetic Causes of Obesity

More than 600 genes, gene markers, and chromosomal regions have been associated with human obesity (1).

Mechanisms of inheritance include the following:

- Single gene mutations
- Autosomal and recessive inheritance
- Candidate genes with obesity as an associated feature
- Linkages with obesity-related phenotypes

The following factors have all been associated with genetic markers (1):

- Body weight
- Body mass index (BMI)
- Fat distribution
- Body composition
- Phenotypes related to energy expenditure
- Waist circumference
- Metabolic syndrome
- Energy and macronutrient intake
- Age at adiposity rebound (1)

The association of obesity with a wide array of genes is not surprising because obesity is intimately associated with energy regulation, a critical factor in survival. Also not surprising is the interaction of genetic susceptibility with the environment. This susceptibility manifests itself in populations who transition from energy-scarce to energy-dense environments either geographically or through successive generations as lifestyles change. The following sections describe a number of genetic syndromes and mutations associated with obesity and give a picture of some of the associated anomalies, which, if seen, should trigger genetic evaluation of the obese child.

GENETIC SYNDROMES AND MUTATIONS

Melanocortin Receptor 4 Mutation

Single gene mutations are a rare cause of obesity. The melanocortin receptor 4 mutation is the most common of these. Leptin stimulates neurons in the arcuate nucleus of the hypothalamus, which express α-melanocyte-stimulating hormone (MSH), and agouti-related peptide, which binds to the MC4R receptor to produce a decrease in food intake (2). Heterozygous missense mutations of MC4R have been found in severely obese children (3).

In a study of obese adults, the prevalence of MC4R mutations was similar in patients who developed obesity in childhood (2.83%) and in those becoming obese in adulthood (2.35%) (4). In a family study with patients who had the onset of obesity before age 10 years, 5.8% had mutations of the MC4R gene. Both homozygous and heterozygous inheritance gave rise to early onset obesity and a pattern of codominance, with the homozygous individuals more obese than the heterozygous individuals. Mutation of MC4R is also associated with severe hyperinsulinemia, which precedes hyperphagia and obesity. Unexpectedly, 32% of the individuals in this study, who were heterozygous, were not obese (5).

Prader-Willi Syndrome

Etiology

Prader-Willi syndrome (PWS) affects about 1 per 10,000 to 1 per 15,000 births. Seventy-three percent of cases result from a deletion of 15q11-q13 from the paternally derived chromosome, involving approximately 4 MB of DNA. The exact gene that causes this syndrome is unknown. Twenty-five percent of cases result from uniparental disomy, which involves inheriting two maternal alleles for chromosome 15 and is associated with advanced maternal age. Rarely, the paternally derived chromosome having maternal DNA methylation can cause Prader-Willi syndrome (4).

Clinical Manifestations

Decreased fetal movement and/or abnormal fetal position at delivery can be a prenatal manifestation of the hypotonia associated with PWS. In the neonate, hypogonadism may be present and can include a hypoplastic scrotum and bilateral or unilateral cryptorchidism. The newborn with PWS can also have poor suck and feeding problems and may present as an infant with failure to thrive. Hyperphagia and food-seeking behavior can become evident between 1 and 6 years of age and are characteristic of this syndrome. The hypothalamic abnormality in PWS results in lack of satiety, and this combined with decreased caloric requirement due to hypotonia, decreased lean body mass, and decreased activity results in obesity (6). Ghrelin, an enteric hunger-producing hormone, is elevated in patients with PWS independent of their BMI (7). Phenotypic features of PWS include a narrow bifrontal facial diameter, almond-shaped palpebral fissure, narrow nasal bridge, and microacria (small hands and feet), with 50% of children reported to have hypopigmentation for the family skin tone. Short stature with growth hormone deficiency is also in the spectrum of findings. Manifestations of hypogonadism include small genitalia, incomplete or delayed pubertal development, and, not uncommonly, infertility. Delayed motor development is always present, with delay of early milestones, language and cognitive delay, and learning disabilities as part of the spectrum. Behavior difficulties are not unusual; temper tantrums, stubborn behavior, obsessive-compulsive tendencies, and difficulty with change are the most common (8). Five percent to 10% of patients may have significant mental illness, including psychosis, bipolar disorder, and obsessive-compulsive disorder. Some special characteristics of this syndrome include having a high threshold for pain, thick viscous saliva, skin picking, high threshold for vomiting, and unusual skill with puzzles (8).

Diagnosis

Classical diagnostic criteria for PWS are listed in Table 14.1 (9). Recently, diagnostic criteria have been expanded to lead to a higher likelihood of diagnosis and earlier intervention. In a review of criteria for diagnosis, children between 2 and 6 years of age with global developmental delay and hypotonia and a history of being a "floppy baby" and having poor feeding with a weak suck would meet criteria for diagnostic testing. By 6 and 12 years of age, children with developmental delay, hyperphagia, and obesity with a similar history of hypotonia in infancy would be candidates for testing. By 13 years and older, evaluation of patients with a similar history, obesity, hyperphagia, and hypogonadotropic hypogonadism would include testing for PWS (6). Genetic testing is performed by DNA methylation test (6). Table 14.2 lists features sufficient to prompt DNA testing.

Treatment

Control of the nutritional environment is crucial in the treatment of PWS. Restricting caloric intake and access to food is the only reliable therapeutic strategy to prevent or limit weight gain. Children with PWS are characterized by a constant drive to find and eat food; they may sneak and hide food, ask others for food, and eat beyond satiety. Parents, family members, and caregivers must be sensitive to these characteristics and work to create a nutritional and activity environment appropriate for these children. Supporting parents and caregivers, educating school regarding portion sizes and access to food, and planning for long-term care are all important aspects of ongoing care.

Case

Initial Presentation

SA is a girl, 3 years and 8 months old, whose mother and aunt bring her to your office for a respiratory illness. As you begin to evaluate her, you note that her weight is 21.2 kg, which is greater than the 95th percentile, and her height is 91.3 cm, which

TABLE 14.1. *Prader-Willi syndrome—diagnostic criteria*

Major criteria (1 point each)
Neonatal and infantile central hypotonia with poor suck, gradually improving
Feeding problems in infancy with need for special feeding techniques and poor weight gain
Excessive or rapid weight gain after 12 months and before age 6, central obesity
Characteristic facial features: dolichocephaly, narrow face, almond-shaped eyes, small-
    appearing mouth, thin upper lip, downturned corner of the mouth (3 or more)
Hypogonadism
Genital hypoplasia
Delayed or incomplete gonadal maturation
Global developmental delay, moderate to mild mental retardation, learning disability
Hyperphagia, food foraging/obsession with food
Deletion of 15q11-13 or maternal disomy

Minor criteria (1/2 point each)
Decreased fetal movement, infantile lethargy, weak cry
Temper tantrums, violent outbursts, OCD, oppositional, rigid manipulative, possessive,
    stubborn, stealing, lying (5 or more)
Sleep disturbance or sleep apnea
Short stature for genetic background
Hypopigmentation for family
Small hands and/or feet
Narrow hands
Esotropia, myopia
Thick, viscous saliva
Speech difficulties
Skin picking

Total points for phenotypic diagnosis
Birth to age 3: 5 total points, including 4 major criteria; 3 to adult: 8 total points, including 5
    major criteria (9)

OCD, obsessive-compulsive disorder.
    Reprinted with permission from Holm VA, Cassidy SB, Butler MG, et al. Prader Willi syn-
drome; consensus diagnostic criteria. *Pediatrics.* 1993;91:398–402.

is less than the 5th percentile, giving her a BMI of 25.4. Her mother tells you that SA was a premature baby with a birth weight of 3 lb 4 oz at 35 weeks. The mother's pregnancy was complicated by gestational diabetes and premature rupture of membranes. The family history is positive for obesity, hypertension, diabetes, thyroid disease, and cardiovascular disease. SA had a complicated neonatal course, which involved respiratory distress syndrome. Mom also noted that a gastrostomy tube had to be placed for poor feeding and hypotonia, but now she is growing well and is "hungry all the time." Over the next few years, SA had repeated episodes of respiratory illness. On physical examination you note that SA has thick saliva, central obesity, and small-appearing hands and feet. You discuss the possibility of a genetic etiology for SA's obesity and developmental delay with the mother and order a methylation study for PWS.

Three Weeks Later

Three weeks later when SA returns to your office, she is feeling much better. You have asked her mother and father to come in to discuss the results of testing. SA

TABLE 14.2. *Features sufficient to prompt DNA testing for Prader-Willi syndrome*

Birth to 2 years
1. Hypotonia with poor suck

2–6 years
1. Hypotonia with history of poor suck
2. Global developmental delay

6–12 years
1. History of hypotonia with poor suck (hypotonia often persists)
2. Global developmental delay
3. Excessive eating (hyperphagia, obsession with food) with central obesity if uncontrolled

13 years through adulthood
1. Cognitive impairment, usually mild mental retardation
2. Excessive eating (hyperphagia, obsession with food) with central obesity if uncontrolled
3. Hypothalamic hypogonadism and/or typical behavior problems (including temper tantrums and obsessive-compulsive features)

Reprinted with permission from Gunay-Aygun M, Schwartz S, Heeger S, O'Riordan MA, Cassiday SB. The changing purpose of Prader-Willi syndrome (clinical diagnostic criteria and proposed revised criteria). *Pediatrics*. 2001;108(5):e92.

does have PWS. You explain the results and describe the syndrome to the parents. You also arrange to have the parents tested for uniparental disomy. They have questions that revolve around SA's development and her eating behavior. You explain about hypothalamic control of eating and the fact that SA, by virtue of having PWS, needs environmental control of access to food to manage her weight. SA's parents are upset but somewhat relieved to find a reason for SA's developmental delay and her food-seeking behavior. You arrange to see the family again in 1 month.

Follow-up Visits

One month later, SA returns, having lost 3 lb. Her parents say they have spoken to other relatives and the daycare she attends and have asked everyone to limit her access to food. They have also eliminated sugar-containing beverages, as you have requested. You urge the parents to keep SA active and ask them to use her stroller as little as possible, encouraging walking and supervised free play. You also ask them to contact SA's school about early developmental programs. You arrange to follow up with her monthly.

Other Single Gene Mutations

Other single gene mutations are listed in Table 14.3.

ALBRIGHT HEREDITARY OSTEODYSTROPHY

Definition

Albright hereditary osteodystrophy is a sex-influenced autosomal dominant syndrome with a female-to-male ratio of 2:1.

TABLE 14.3. *Single gene mutations*

- Leptin receptor gene *1p31*
  Early-onset morbid obesity; homozygous patients have no pubertal development and decreased secretion of growth hormone and thyrotropin (10)

- *PCSKI* (protein convertase subtilisin/kexin type I) gene 5q15-q21
  Extreme childhood obesity, abnormal glucose homeostasis, hypogonadotropic hypogonadism, hypercortisolism, elevated plasma proinsulin and POMC concentrations but very low insulin levels, suggestive of defective prohormone processing (11)

- 17q22-q24 growth hormone deficiency
  Delayed skeletal maturation and height retardation, truncal obesity, delayed secondary dentition, high-pitched voice, and delayed puberty (12)

- *MC4R* (melanocortin 4 receptor) 18q21.3 (see text)

- Prader-Willi syndrome 15q11-q13 (see text)

- Ulnar mammary syndrome 12q24.1
  Ulnar finger and fibular toe ray defects; delayed growth and onset of puberty, obesity, and hypogenitalism and diminished sexual activity; and hypoplasia of nipples and apocrine glands with subsequent diminished ability to perspire (13)

POMC, pro-opiomelanocortin.

Clinical Manifestations

One of the earliest identifiable features of the syndrome is early onset of hypocalcemia, with 80% of affected children having hypocalcemia in the first or second year of life. Other features in addition to obesity and hypocalcemia include the following:

- Short stature
- Brachydactyly
- Ectopic calcifications
- Mental retardation
- Pseudohypoparathyroidism

Short stature is characterized by generalized shortening of the extremities and cone-shaped, absent, or prematurely closed epiphysis (14).

AUTOSOMAL RECESSIVE DISORDERS

Bardet-Biedl Syndrome

Definition

Bardet-Biedl syndrome is a heterogeneous autosomal recessive disorder associated with five separate genetic loci: 11q13 (BBS1), 16q21 (BBS2), 3p12-13 (BBS3), 15q22.22-q23 (BBS4), and 2q31 (BBS5).

Clinical Manifestations

Characteristics of this syndrome include the following:

- Obesity
- Mild mental retardation
- Pigmentary retinopathy with loss of visual acuity and dark adaptation
- Polydactyly
- Hypogonadism
- Renal dysfunction

Symptoms are variable among subgroups: 90% of adults in all groups are above the 90th percentile for weight, children younger than 10 years may be below the 90th percentile in some subtypes, and obligate heterozygotes are reported to have increased incidence of obesity, diabetes, hypertension, and renal disease. Pigmentary retinopathy in this syndrome is associated with abnormal electroretinograms in infancy, degeneration of retinal photoreceptors affecting cones and rods, and progressive loss of visual acuity and dark-adapted sensitivity. Visual acuity decreases to the 20/100 range by about 11 to 12 years, and 93% of patients older than 30 years are legally blind. There is universal infertility in males with hypogonadism, poorly developed secondary sexual characteristics, and primary testicular pathology. Hypothalamic-pituitary and ovarian dysfunction is present in females; secondary sexual characteristics are normal, but there is an increased rate of structural genitourinary abnormalities. Ninety percent of patients have renal involvement, which is characterized by heterogeneous parenchymal lesions, distal tubular dysfunction, and glomerular disease (15).

Other Autosomal Recessive Disorders

Other autosomal recessive disorders are listed in Table 14.4.

X-LINKED DISORDERS

Obesity has also been associated with X-linked disorders (Table 14.5).

TABLE 14.4. *Autosomal recessive disorders*

- Alstrom's syndrome 2p14-p13
  Early childhood retinopathy, progressive sensorineural hearing loss, truncal obesity, and acanthosis nigricans (16)
- Bardet-Biedl syndrome 1 11q13 (see text)
- Bardet-Biedl syndrome 2 16q21 (see text)
- Bardet-Biedl syndrome 3 3p13-p12 (see text)
- Bardet-Biedl syndrome 4 15q22.3-q23 9 (see text)
- Cohen's syndrome 8q22-q23
  Developmental delay, microcephaly, truncal obesity with slender extremities, sociable behavior, joint hypermobility, high myopia and/or retinal dystrophy, and neutropenia. Patients fulfilling 6 or more criteria likely to have true Cohen's syndrome (17)

TABLE 14.5. *X-linked disorders*

- Mehmo's syndrome Xp22.13-p21.1
  Mental retardation, epileptic seizures, hypogonadism and hypogenitalism, microcephaly, and obesity with death in childhood (18)
- Wilson-Turner syndrome Xp21.1q22
  Mental retardation, obesity, gynecomastia, speech difficulties, emotional lability, tapering fingers, and small feet (19)

REFERENCES

1. Perusse L, Rankinen T, Zuberi A, Chagnon YC, Wesinagel AJ, Argyropoulos G, Waltsm B, Snyder EE, Bouchard C. The human obesity gene map; the 2004 update. *Obes Res.* 2005;13(3):381–490.
2. Lubrano-Berthelier C, Le Stunff C, Bougneres P, Vaisse C. A homozygous null mutation delineates the role of the melanocortin 4 receptor in humans. *J Clin Endocrinol Metab.* 2004;89(5):2028–2032.
3. Dubern B, Clement K, Pelloux V, Froguel P, Girardet JP, Guy-Grand B, Tounian P. Mutational analysis of melanocortin-4 receptor, agouti-related protein and alpha melanocyte stimulating hormone genes in severely obese children. *J Pediatr.* 2001;139(2):204–209.
4. Lubrano-Berthelier C, Dubern B, Lacorte JM, Picard F, Shapiro A, Zang S, Bertais S, Hercberg S, Basdevant A, Clement K, Vaisse C. Melanocortin 4 receptor mutations in a large cohort of severely obese adults; prevalence, functional classification, genotype-phenotype relationship and lack of association with binge eating. *J Clin Endocrinol Metab.* 2006;91(5):1811–1818.
5. Farooqi IS, Keogh JM, Yeo GS, Lank EJ, Cheetham T, O'Rahilly S Clinical spectrum of obesity and mutations in the melanocortin 4 receptor gene. *N Engl J Med.* 2003;348(12):1085–1095.
6. Gunay-Aygun M, Schwartz S, Heeger S, O'Riordan MA, Cassiday SB. The changing purpose of Prader-Willi syndrome (clinical diagnostic criteria and proposed revised criteria). *Pediatrics.* 2001;108(5):e92.
7. Cummings DE, Clement K, Parnell JQ, Vaisse C, Foster KE, Frayo RS, Schwartz MW, Basdevant A, Weigle DS. Elevated plasma ghrelin levels in Prader-Willi syndrome. *Nat Med.* 2002;8(7):643–644.
8. Cassidy SB. Prader-Willi syndrome. *J Med Genet.* 1997;34(11):917–923.
9. Holm VA, Cassidy SB, Butler MG, Hanchett JM, Greenswag LR, Whitman BY, Greenberg F. Prader Willi syndrome: consensus diagnostic criteria. *Pediatrics.* 1993;91(2):398–402.
10. Clement K, Vaisse C, Lahlou N, Cabrol S, Pelloux V, Cassuto D, Gourmelen M, Dina C, Chambaz J, Lacorte JM, Basdevant A, Bougneres P, Lebouc Y, Froguel P, Guy-Grand B. A mutation in the human leptin receptor gene causes obesity and pituitary dysfunction. *Nature.* 1998;392(6674):398–401.
11. O'Rahilly S, Gray H, Humphreys PJ, Krook A, Polonsky KS, White A, Gibson S, Taylor K, Carr, C. Brief report: impaired processing of prohormones associated with abnormalities of glucose homeostasis and adrenal function. *N Engl J Med.* 1995;333(21):1386–1390.
12. Rimoin DL, Phillips JA. Genetic disorders of the pituitary gland. In: Rimoin DL, Connor JM, Pyeritz RE, eds. *Principles and practice of medical genetics,* Vol. I, 3rd ed. New York: Churchill Livingstone; 1997:1331–1364.
13. Schinzel A, Illig R, Prader A. The ulnar-mammary syndrome: an autosomal dominant pleiotropic gene. *Clin Genet.* 1987;32:160–168. Erratum: *Clin Genet.* 1987;32:425.
14. Ong KK, Amin R, Dunger DB. Pseudohypoparathyroidism—another monogenic obesity syndrome. *Clin Endocrinol (Oxf).* 2000;52(3):389–391.
15. Green JS, Parfrey PS, Harnett JD, Farid NR, Cramer BC, Johnson G, Heath O, McManamon PJ, O'Leary E, Pryse-Phillips W, The cardinal manifestations of Bardet-Biedl syndrome, a form of Laurence-Moon-Biedl syndrome. *N Engl J Med.* 1989;321(15):1002–1009.
16. Marshall JD, Ludman MD, Shea SE, Salisbury SR, Willi SM, LaRoche RG, Nishina PM. Genealogy, natural history, and phenotype of Alstrom syndrome in a large Acadian kindred and three additional families. *Am J Med Genet.* 1997;73:150–161.
17. Kolehmainen J, Wilkinson R, Lehesjoki, AE, Chandler K, Kivitie-Kallio S, Clayton-Smith J, Traskelin AL, Waris L, Saarinen A, Khan J, Gross-Tsur V, Traboulsi EI, Warburg M, Fryns JP, Norio R, Black GC, Manson FD. Delineation of Cohen syndrome following a large-scale genotype-phenotype screen. *Am J Hum Genet.* 2004;75(1):122–127.
18. Steinmuller R, Steinberger D, Muller U. MEHMO (mental retardation, epileptic seizures, hypogonadism and -genitalism, microcephaly, obesity), a novel syndrome: assignment of disease locus to Xp21.1-p22.13. *Eur J Hum Genet.* 1998;6(3):201–206.
19. Wilson M, Mulley J, Gedeon A, Robinson H, Turner, G. New X-linked syndrome of mental retardation, gynecomastia, and obesity is linked to DXS255. *Am J Med Genet.* 1991;40(4):406–413.

15

Acute Obesity-Related Emergencies

Obesity is a chronic disease; however, obesity-related life-threatening emergencies can occur and must be considered as part of the obesity spectrum of care. Both hyperglycemic hyperosmolar state (HHS) and diabetic ketoacidosis (DKA) can be life-threatening presentations of type 2 diabetes. Pulmonary emboli and cardiomyopathy of obesity are rare but emergent cardiovascular complications of obesity. Each of these complications both illustrates the severity of obesity and highlights aspects of pathophysiology that can occur in the pediatric age group.

HYPERGLYCEMIC HYPEROSMOLAR STATE

State of the Problem

Cases of HHS have now been reported in adolescents with type 2 diabetes. Morales and Rosenbloom (1) described seven obese African American teenagers who were considered to have died of DKA. On review, these adolescents were found instead to have had HHS.

Etiology

Hyperglycemia in the absence of ketosis can occur in diabetic patients with type 2 diabetes. Relative insulin deficiency develops in the obese patient as insulin resistance increases and beta cell function declines. Loss of suppression of hepatic glucose production occurs, with attendant hyperglycemia. However, enough insulin function may remain to allow suppression of ketosis and lipolysis (2). The initial event in HHS is glycosuric diuresis with glycosuria, impeding the concentrating ability of the kidney and increasing water loss (3). The decreased glomerular filtration rate causes glucose to increase with excess water loss over the sodium loss, leading to hyperosmolarity. Insulin is present but, because of greater insulin resistance, cannot reduce the serum glucose (4). It is important to be alert for signs and symptoms of type 2 diabetes in obese children and adolescents and to be able to recognize HHS on presentation.

Clinical Manifestations

A review of 190 children and adolescents with type 2 diabetes presenting over a 5-year period found the frequency of HHS to be 3.7%. All seven patients diagnosed with HHS were African American children with an average age of 13.3 years (10–16 years) whose initial presentation with type 2 diabetes was with an episode of HHS. The mean body mass index (BMI) was 32.7 kg/m². The mean serum osmolality was 393 mOsm/L, and the mean blood glucose was 1,604 mg/dL. One patient died (5). Death in HHS has been reported to occur from hypovolemic shock and rhabdomyolysis with multisystem organ failure (6). An adolescent patient presenting with HHS has been reported dying on the sixth day of hospitalization from a massive pulmonary embolism (PE) (7).

Patients have presented to medical care with symptoms of vomiting, abdominal pain, dizziness, weakness, polyuria/polydipsia, weight loss, and diarrhea prior to death, which may not be linked to the presentation of type 2 diabetes unless there is a high index of suspicion.

Diagnostic criteria for HHS include the following:

- Plasma glucose greater than 600 mg/dL
- Serum carbon dioxide greater than 15 mmol/L
- Small or absent ketonuria
- Ketonemia
- Serum osmolality greater than 320 mOsm/kg
- Stupor or coma (1,8)

Mortality rates of 14% in adolescents presenting with HHS have been reported (5). A fatal malignant hyperthermia syndrome with rhabdomyolysis and hyperpyrexia has been described in obese adolescent males with HHS (9).

DIABETIC KETOACIDOSIS

State of the Problem

Type 2 diabetes can present with DKA. If basal insulin sensitivity is low, as it is in obese patients with insulin resistance, there is increasing susceptibility to relative insulin deficiency.

Etiology

The cause of DKA in type 2 diabetes is hyperglycemia with relative insulin deficiency, producing increased lipolysis and release of free fatty acids, as well as ketonemia and ketonuria (Fig. 15.1).

Epidemiology

In a series of patients aged 9 to 18 years presenting with DKA, there was a 13% prevalence of patients with type 2 diabetes (10). DKA has been reported in a

Diabetic Ketoacidosis

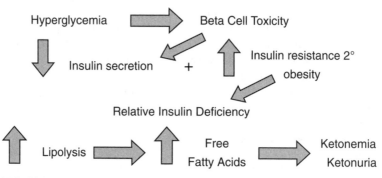

FIG. 15.1. Diabetic ketoacidosis.

13-year-old boy with Prader-Willi syndrome and nonalcoholic steatohepatitis (NASH) 1 month after beginning growth hormone therapy. The hyperglycemia resolved 2 months after growth hormone therapy discontinuation, but the patient developed type 2 diabetes 6 months later with weight gain (11).

Pathophysiology

The pathophysiology of DKA results from relative insulin deficiency and elevated levels of counter-regulatory hormones. When insulin is deficient, increased glucagon, catecholamines, and cortisol stimulate hepatic glucose production by increasing glycogenolysis and gluconeogenesis. The rise in cortisol increases protein breakdown and the availability of amino acid precursors for gluconeogenesis. Low insulin and high catecholamine levels reduce peripheral uptake of glucose. These processes result in hyperglycemia, which causes glycosuria, osmotic diuresis and dehydration, and decreased renal perfusion.

In DKA, hormone-sensitive lipase is activated in a state of low insulin availability. Elevated catecholamines, cortisol, and growth hormone cause the breaking down of triglyceride and the release of free fatty acids. Free fatty acids are converted to ketones in the liver and are released, causing ketonemia. An increase in glucagon causes increases in acyl coenzyme A, a substrate for synthesis of hydroxybutyric acid and acetoacetic acid, the main contributors to acidosis (12).

Diagnosis

Diagnostic criteria for DKA are blood glucose greater than 11 mmol/L (normal 4.2–6.4 mmol/L), venous pH less than 7.3 (normal 7.35–7.45), and/or serum bicarbonate less than 15 mmol/L. There is associated glycosuria, ketonuria, and ketonemia (12,13).

Diagnosis, monitoring, and treatment have recently been reviewed (13). Success of treatment depends on correction of dehydration to restore renal perfusion and to correct hyperglycemia, ketoacidosis, and electrolyte deficits (12,13).

PULMONARY EMBOLISM

State of the Problem

Pulmonary embolism is more common in adult obese patients than in the pediatric age group. Symptoms of PE include the following:

- Dyspnea
- Chest pain
- Hypoxia
- Hemoptysis

In a study of PE in adolescents, adolescents were more likely to have a normal chest radiograph, less likely to be tachypneic, and less likely to have an abnormal chest examination than adults. PE should be considered for "any adolescent who presents with unexplained pleuritic chest pain, dyspnea, or hypoxemia, particularly in the presence of risk factors or supportive exam findings" (14).

Epidemiology

The incidence of PE increases with age in adults. In adults, antithrombotic drugs are the mainstay of prevention and treatment (15). A review of National Hospital Survey Data showed a relative risk of deep venous thrombosis of 2.5 in obese compared with normal weight adults and a relative risk of developing a PE of 2.21. Females and patients younger than 40 years were at somewhat greater risk (16).

Pathophysiology

Obesity and the associated metabolic disorders may increase the risk of venous thrombosis by altering the balance between thrombotic and thrombolytic activity. Ob/ob leptin-deficient mice have a decreased thrombotic response and experience a lower rate of venous thrombosis and PE after injury than normal mice (17). Sixty percent of normal mice pretreated with a leptin-neutralizing antibody survived otherwise lethal venous thrombosis and PE. Obese humans have an excess of leptin and leptin resistance, which may play a role in their increased risk of thrombosis (17).

Etiology

The major factors contributing to PE in adults are as follows (18):

- Heart disease
- Cancer
- Obesity

- Acute paraplegia
- Trauma
- Prior history of venous thromboembolism
- Pregnancy
- Use of oral contraceptives
- Inflammatory bowel disease
- Coagulation disorders (19)
- Obstructive sleep apnea syndrome (19)

In adults, risk of deep vein thrombosis is doubled in obese patients (20). Both obesity and trauma are risk factors for deep vein thrombosis and PE and prophylactic anticoagulation has been recommended as treatment for adult trauma patients who are obese (21).

PE can be a complication of bariatric surgery and the most common cause of unexpected death in the morbidly obese patient (22). PE has been reported in adolescents following gastric bypass surgery (23). PE can also be a complication of orthopedic surgery. Adults undergoing hip fracture surgery who were receiving prophylaxis had mortality and fatal PE rates of 3.2% (2.8% to 3.6%) and 0.30% (0% to 0.61%) (24). Prevention of deep venous thrombosis and PE includes the reduction of obesity and inactivity and the cessation of cigarette smoking.

CARDIOMYOPATHY OF OBESITY

State of the Problem

BMI is positively correlated with increased right-sided heart pressures, cardiac output, pulmonary vascular resistance index, and systolic blood pressure in adults with congestive heart failure. One study found that obese patients had higher right-sided heart pressures, cardiac output, and pulmonary vascular resistance index when compared with a group of lean patients having a similar degree of cardiomyopathy (25).

Etiology

The cardiomyopathy of obesity is thought to result from high metabolic activity of excessive fat, which increases total blood volume and cardiac output, resulting in left ventricular dysfunction. Left ventricular wall stress increases, causing dilation and compensatory left ventricular hypertrophy and diastolic dysfunction, which results in heart failure (Fig. 15.2). Right ventricular dysfunction can be exacerbated by pulmonary hypertension due to upper airway obstruction (26).

In obese Zucker mice, excess lipid accumulates in the myocardium, which may cause a "lipotoxic" cardiomyopathy (27). Recent imaging studies in humans have shown that myocardial lipid content increases with the degree of adiposity (28).

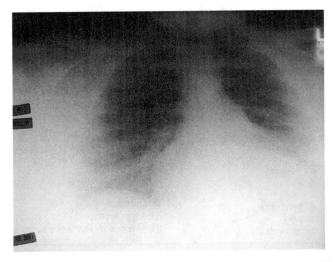

FIG. 15.2. A 17-year-old patient with biventricular cardiac failure and cardiomyopathy of obesity.

ISSUES IN INTENSIVE CARE OF THE OBESE CHILD AND ADOLESCENT

As the epidemic of obesity and morbid obesity increases in the pediatric age group, obesity-related comorbidities are becoming more common and need to be identified in any hospitalized obese patient (Table 15.1). Signs and symptoms suggestive of these comorbidities should be promptly investigated.

Issues related to proper-sized equipment and accurate drug dosing should be addressed on an individual basis for each obese patient.

Cardiorespiratory Considerations

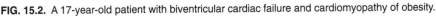

Pulmonary mechanics are altered by obesity.

Chest wall compliance is reduced, and full anterior excursion is hampered (29). Forced expiratory reserve volume in one second (FEV_1), forced expiratory flow between 25% and 75% of forced vital capacity (FEV_{25-75}), and diffusing capacity for carbon monoxide have all been found to be reduced in obese children (30).

Upper airway obstruction should be identified in any hospitalized obese patient with symptoms of snoring, apnea, history of orthopnea, daytime tiredness, poor school performance or executive functioning, or family history of upper airway obstruction. Bilevel airway pressure (BiPAP) or continuous positive airway pressure

TABLE 15.1. *Obesity-related comorbidities*

Respiratory Asthma Sleep apnea/upper airway obstruction Restrictive lung disease	**Genetic syndromes** Prader-Willi syndrome Bardet-Biedl syndrome Alstrom's syndrome
Cardiovascular Hypertension Dyslipidemia Left ventricular dysfunction/cardiomyopathy Reduced level of deconditioning	**Neurologic** Headaches due to pseudotumor cerebri Hypothalamic dysfunction/injury
Metabolic Impaired glucose tolerance Insulin resistance Type 2 diabetes Polycystic ovarian syndrome Premature adrenarche Pubertal acceleration or delay	**Gastrointestinal** Nonalcoholic fatty liver disease Nonalcoholic steatohepatitis Cirrhosis Gastroesophageal reflux **Musculoskeletal** Blount's disease Slipped capital femoral epiphysis

(CPAP) should be prescribed if used at home; a sleep study should be performed if symptoms are present prior to elective hospitalization so proper respiratory support can be provided. In a series of 14 obese patients undergoing tonsilloadenoidectomy for obstructive sleep apnea, 2 patients required overnight BiPAP for oxygen desaturation, 1 patient required prolonged intubation, and 3 patients required supplemental oxygen (31). Prior history of asthma, asthma exacerbations, and seriousness of intervention needed should be ascertained in the obese child admitted to the hospital. Hospitalization may present an opportunity to optimize asthma therapy in this population. Restrictive lung disease is a component of the respiratory derangements in obesity, and because of this, postoperative attention to pulmonary toilet may be especially important in these patients.

Respiratory issues need to be anticipated in morbidly obese patients, with adequate respiratory support provided in the immediate postoperative period (32).

Metabolic Considerations

Severe illness may exacerbate hyperglycemia. In adults in an intensive care unit, hyperglycemia was common and associated with adequacy of glucose regulation prior to the acute hospitalization. This relationship with prior glucose control held true even in nondiabetic patients. Treatment with steroids, norepinephrine, and carbohydrate administration contributed to hyperglycemia (33).

Adult surgical patients in a surgical intensive care setting receiving mechanical ventilation were randomized to receive usual care or intensive control of blood glucose levels between 80 and 110 mg/dL. Mortality in the intensive control group was half (4.6% vs. 8.0%) of that in the usual care group. Improved outcome was due to decreased incidence of sepsis in patients with longer term stays in the intensive care unit. Intensive insulin therapy also prevented acute renal failure (34).

In another study, morbidly obese (BMI >40 kg/m^2) and normal weight adults admitted to an intensive care unit were compared regarding outcomes. Sixty-one percent of the obese patients required mechanical ventilation versus 46% of normal weight patients. Length of mechanical ventilation and stay in the intensive care unit was increased, and mortality was almost double that of the normal weight patients (30% vs. 17%). Multiorgan failure, respiratory failure, and left ventricular dysfunction were associated with the increased mortality (35). Children and adolescents with morbid obesity will have the normal range of infections, trauma, and metabolic diseases expected in a pediatric population. Few studies have been performed that assess the impact of obesity on children in the hospital and intensive care unit.

Individualized assessment and planning are critical for any obese child undergoing hospitalization.

REFERENCES

1. Morales AE, Rosenbloom AL. Death caused by hyperglycemic hyperosmolar state at the onset of type 2 diabetes. *J Pediatr.* 2004;144(2):270–273.
2. Glaser N. Pediatric diabetic ketoacidosis and hyperglycemic hyperosmolar state. *Pediatr Clin North Am.* 2005;52(6):1611–1635.
3. Wachtel T, Stillman R, Lamberton P. Predisposing factors of diabetic hyperosmolar state. *Arch Intern Med.* 1987;147(3):499–501.
4. Stoner GD. Hyperosmolar hyperglycemic state. *Am Fam Physician.* 2005; 71(9): 1723–1730.
5. Fourtner SH, Weinzimer SA, Levitt Katz LE. Hyperglycemic hyperosmolar non-ketotic syndrome in children with type 2 diabetes. *Pediatr Diabetes.* 2005;6(3):129–135.
6. Carchman RM, Dechert-Zeger M, Calikogluc AS, Hasrris BD. A new challenge in pediatric obesity; pediatric hyperglycemic hyperosmolar syndrome. *Pediatr Crit Care Med.* 2005;6(1):20–24.
7. Bhowmick SK, Levens KL, Rettig KR. Hyperosmolar hyperglycemic crisis: an acute life-threatening event in children and adolescents with type 2 diabetes mellitus. *Endocr Pract.* 2005;11(1):23–29.
8. Rubin HM, Kramer R, Drash A. Hyperosmolarity complicating diabetes mellitus in childhood. *J Pediatr.* 1969:74:177–186.
9. Hollander A, Olney R, Blackett P, Marshall BA. Fatal malignant hyperthermia like syndrome with rhabdomyolysis complicating the presentation of diabetes mellitus in adolescent males. *Pediatrics.* 2003;111(6Pt1):1447–1452.
10. Sapru A, Gitelman SE, Bhatia SK, Bubin RF, Newman TB, Flori H. Prevalence and characteristics of type 2 diabetes mellitus in 9-18 year old children with diabetic ketoacidosis. *J Pediatr Endocrinol Metab.* 2005;18(9):865–872.
11. Yigit S, Estrada E, Hyams J, Rosengren J. Diabetic ketoacidosis secondary to growth hormone treatment in a boy with Prader-Willi syndrome and steatohepatitis. *J Pediatr Endocrinol.* 2004;17(3):361–364.
12. Chiasson JL, Aris-Jilwan N, Belanger R, Bertrand S. Diagnosis and treatment of diabetic ketoacidosis and the hyperglycemic hyperosmolar state. *CMAJ.* 2003;168(7):1–19.
13. Dunger DB, Sperling MA, Acerini CL, Bohn DJ, Daneman D, Glaser NS, Hanas R, Hintz RL, Levitsky LL, Savage MO, Tasker RC, Wolfsdorf JI . European Society for Pediatric Endocrinology/Lawson Wilkins Pediatric Endocrine Society consensus statement on diabetic ketoacidosis in children and adolescents. *Pediatrics.* 2004;113:e133–e140.

14. Bernstein D, Coupey S, Schonberg K. Pulmonary embolism in adolescents. *Am J Dis Child.* 1986;140(7):667–671.
15. Motsch J, Walther A, Bock M, Bottiger BW. Update in the prevention and treatment of deep vein thrombosis and pulmonary embolism. *Curr Opin Anaesthesiol.* 2006;19(1):52–58.
16. Stein PD, Beemath A, Olson RE. Obesity as a risk factor in venous thromboembolism. *Am J Med.* 2005;118(9):978–980.
17. Konstantinides S, Schafer K, Neels JG, Dellas C, Loskutoff DJ. Inhibition of endogenous leptin protects mice from arterial and venous thrombosis. *Arterioscler Thromb Vasc Biol.* 2004;24(11):2196–2201.
18. Coon WW. Risk factors in pulmonary embolism. *Surg Gynecol Obstet.* 1976;143:385–390.
19. Koenig SM. Pulmonary complications of obesity. *Am J Med Sci.* 2001;321(4):249–279.
20. Abdollahi M, Cushman M, Rosendaal FR. Obesity: risk of venous thrombosis and the interaction with coagulation factor levels and oral contraceptive use. *Thromb Haemost.* 2003;89(3):493–498.
21. Frezza EE, Chiriva-Internati M. Venous thromboembolism in morbid obesity and trauma. A review of literature. *Minerva Chir.* 2005;60(5):391–399.
22. Pulipati RC, Lazzaro RS, Macura J, Savel RH. Successful thrombolysis of submassive pulmonary embolism after bariatric surgery: expanding indication and addressing the controversies. *Obes Surg.* 2003;13(5):792–796.
23. Sugerman HJ, Sugerman EL, DeMaria EJ, Kellum JM, Kennedy C, Mowery Y, Wolfe LG. Bariatric surgery for severely obese adolescents. *J Gastrointest Surg.* 2003;7(1):102–107.
24. Dahl OE, Carpini JA, Colwell CS, Froswtick SP, Haas S, Hull RD, Laporte S, Stein PD. Fatal vascular outcomes following major orthopedic surgery. *Thromb Hemost.* 2005;93(5):860–866.
25. Kasper EK, Hrubn RH, Baughman KL. Cardiomyopathy of obesity a clinical pathologic evaluation of 43 obese patients with heart failure. *Am J Cardiol.* 1992;70(9):921–924.
26. Alpert MA. Obesity: cardiomyopathy pathophysiology and evolution of the clinical syndrome. *Am J Med Sci.* 2001;321(4):225–236.
27. Wang MY, Unger RH. Role of PP2C in cardiac lipid accumulation in obese rodents and its prevention by troglitazone. *Am J Physiol Endocrinol Metab.* 2005;288(1):e216–e221.
28. McGavock JM, Victor RG, Unger RH, Szczepaniak LS; American College of Physicians and the American Physiological Society. Adiposity of the heart, revisited. *Ann Intern Med.* 2006;144(7):517–524.
29. Brenn BR. Anesthesia for pediatric obesity. *Anesthesiol Clin North Am.* 2005;23(4):745–764.
30. Inselman LS, Milanese A, Deurloo A. Effect of obesity on pulmonary function in children. *Pediatr Pulmonol.* 1993;16(2):130–137.
31. Spector A, Scheid S, Hassink S, Deutsch ES, Reilly JS, Cook SP. Adenotonsillectomy in the morbidly obese child. *Int J Pediatr Otorhinolaryngol.* 2003;67(4):359–364.
32. Tseng CH, Chen C, Wong CH, Wong SY, Wong KM. Anesthesia for pediatric patients with Prader-Willi syndrome: report of two cases. *Chang Gung Med J.* 2003;26(6):453–457.
33. Cely CM, Arora P, Quartin AA, Kett DH, Schein RMH. Relationship of baseline glucose homeostasis to hyperglycemia during medical critical illness. *Chest.* 2004;126(3):879–887.
34. Van den Berghe G, Wouters P, Weekers F, Verwaest C, Bruyninckx F, Schetz M, Vlasselaers D, Ferdinande P, Lauwers P, Bouillon R. Intensive insulin therapy in critically ill patients. *N Engl J Med.* 2001;345:1359–1367.
35. El-Solh A, Sikka P, Bozkanat E, Jaafar W, Davies J. Morbid obesity in the medical ICU. *Chest.* 2001;120:1989–1997.

16

Practice Management Strategies for Obesity

When 25% to 50% of children and adolescents are affected by overweight or obesity, every clinician caring for children will need to develop strategies for dealing with obesity prevention, identification, early intervention, and treatment. Although obesity treatment without question needs to be individualized, there are clear practice-based strategies that will help in prevention, identification, and early intervention.

Factors of time and cost have to be considered as practice patterns change to meet the demands of caring for the obese child. In addition, physicians, nurses, and ancillary staff will need to be educated, to allow incorporation of this "new work" into day-to-day practice management.

DEFINITIONS

- **Underweight**—Body mass index (BMI) less than the 5th percentile
- **Normal weight**—BMI between the 5th and 85th percentiles
- **Overweight**—BMI between the 85th and 95th percentiles
- **Obese**—BMI greater than the 95th percentile

PREVENTION

> One should monitor height, weight, and BMI for all children at every encounter.

Primary prevention of obesity is a goal shared by everyone in pediatric health care. From the beginning, achieving energy balance with appropriate growth in a setting of optimal nutrition, activity, and inactivity should be the goal. With this goal in mind, the following principles could be followed as a way to address obesity prevention in practice.

The practice of monitoring growth beginning at birth, plotting weight-for-length charts for infants (Figs. 16.1 and 16.2) and BMI charts for children older than 2 years

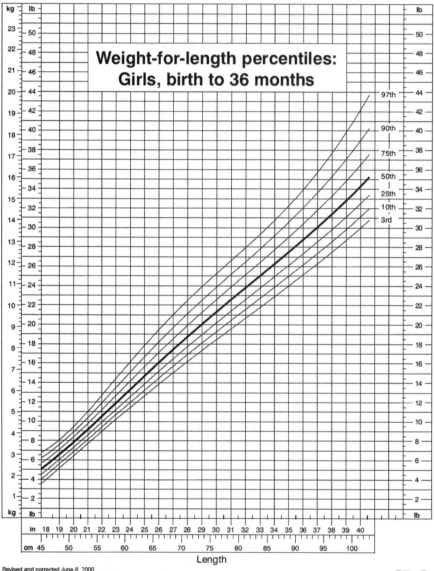

FIG. 16.1. Weight-for-length percentiles: girls 0 to 36 months. (Developed by the National Center for Health Statistics in collaboration with the National Center for Chronic Disease.)

(Figs. 16.3 and 16.4), and sharing these measurements with families is a good way to introduce your concern about optimal growth as well as to begin to discuss energy balance.

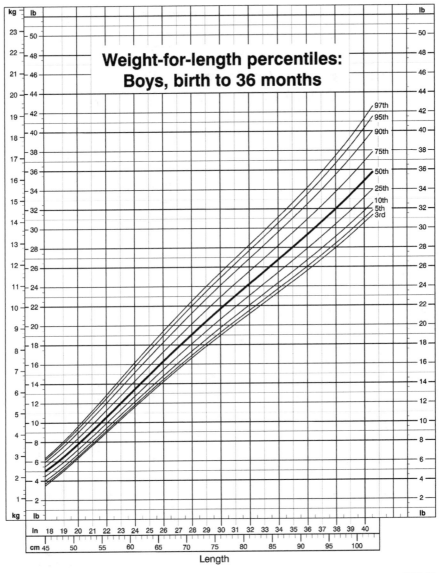

CDC Growth Charts: United States

Weight-for-length percentiles: Boys, birth to 36 months

Length

Revised and corrected June 5, 2000.
SOURCE: Developed by the National Center for Health Statistics in collaboration with the National Center for Chronic Disease Prevention and Health Promotion (2000).

FIG. 16.2. Weight-for-length percentiles: boys 0 to 36 months. (Developed by the National Center for Health Statistics in collaboration with the National Center for Chronic Disease.)

Routine recommended preventive care screening should be performed for children following a normal growth trajectory with no obesity or obesity comorbidity risk factors. Periodic review of family history, growth trajectory, and nutrition and activity habits should be incorporated into these well care visits.

CDC Growth Charts: United States

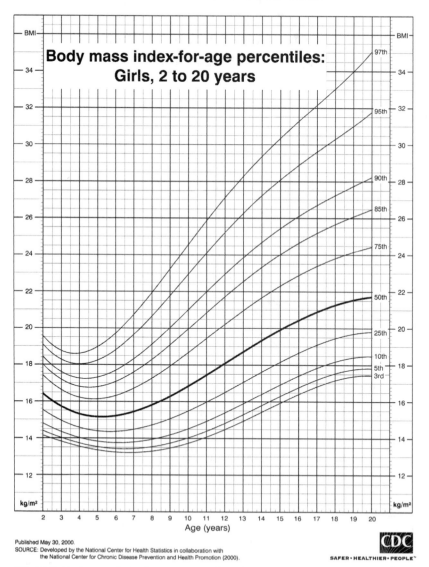

FIG. 16.3. Body mass index-for-age percentiles: girls 2 to 20 years. (Developed by the National Center for Health Statistics in collaboration with the National Center for Chronic Disease.)

Opportunities to plot height, weight, and BMI should be taken advantage of at all possible visits, reinforcing good nutrition and activity habits.

CDC Growth Charts: United States

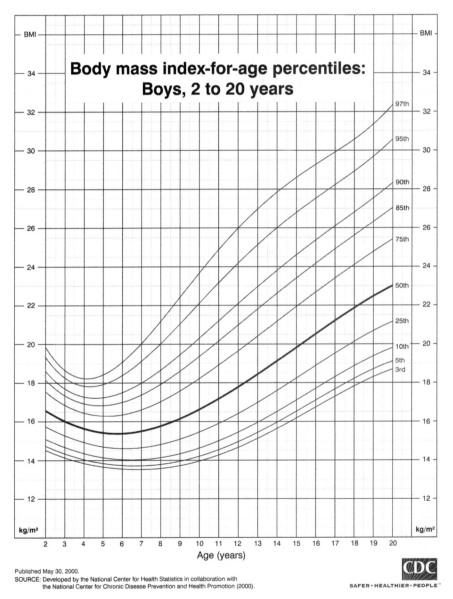

Published May 30, 2000.
SOURCE: Developed by the National Center for Health Statistics in collaboration with the National Center for Chronic Disease Prevention and Health Promotion (2000).

SAFER·HEALTHIER·PEOPLE™

FIG. 16.4. Body mass index-for-age percentiles: boys 2 to 20 years. (Developed by the National Center for Health Statistics in collaboration with the National Center for Chronic Disease.)

Weight and length/height (stature) charts are given in Figures 16.5 through 16.12.

Text continued on page 188.

CDC Growth Charts: United States

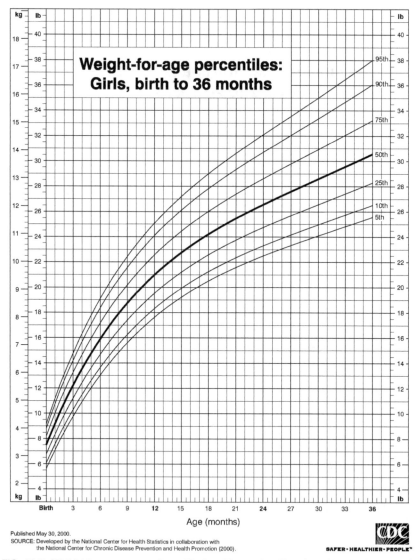

Weight-for-age percentiles: Girls, birth to 36 months

Published May 30, 2000.
SOURCE: Developed by the National Center for Health Statistics in collaboration with the National Center for Chronic Disease Prevention and Health Promotion (2000).

FIG. 16.5. Weight-for-age percentiles: girls 0 to 36 months. (Developed by the National Center for Health Statistics in collaboration with the National Center for Chronic Disease.)

CDC Growth Charts: United States

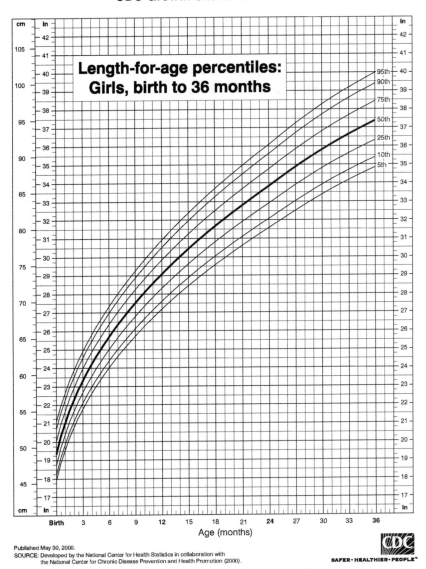

Length-for-age percentiles: Girls, birth to 36 months

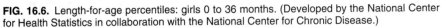

Published May 30, 2000.
SOURCE: Developed by the National Center for Health Statistics in collaboration with the National Center for Chronic Disease Prevention and Health Promotion (2000).

SAFER·HEALTHIER·PEOPLE™

FIG. 16.6. Length-for-age percentiles: girls 0 to 36 months. (Developed by the National Center for Health Statistics in collaboration with the National Center for Chronic Disease.)

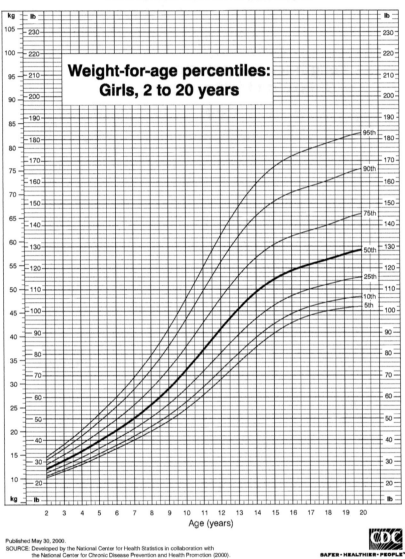

FIG. 16.7. Weight-for-age percentiles: girls 2 to 20 years. (Developed by the National Center for Health Statistics in collaboration with the National Center for Chronic Disease.)

CDC Growth Charts: United States

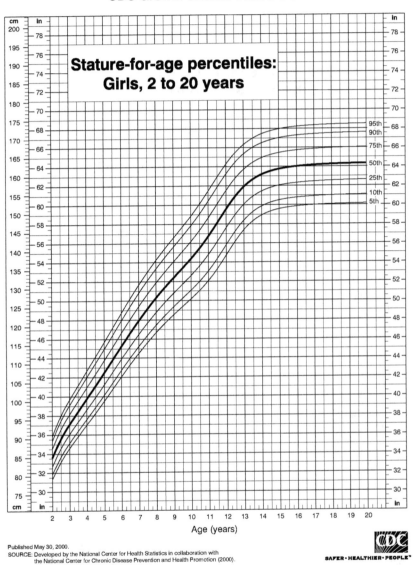

Stature-for-age percentiles: Girls, 2 to 20 years

Published May 30, 2000.
SOURCE: Developed by the National Center for Health Statistics in collaboration with
the National Center for Chronic Disease Prevention and Health Promotion (2000).

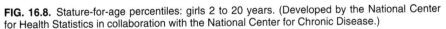

FIG. 16.8. Stature-for-age percentiles: girls 2 to 20 years. (Developed by the National Center for Health Statistics in collaboration with the National Center for Chronic Disease.)

CDC Growth Charts: United States

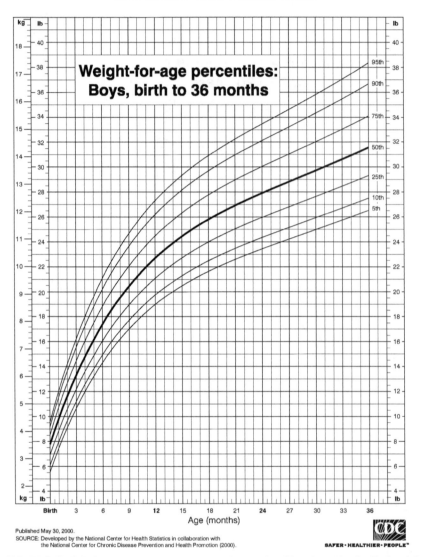

FIG. 16.9. Weight-for-age percentiles: boys 0 to 36 months. (Developed by the National Center for Health Statistics in collaboration with the National Center for Chronic Disease.)

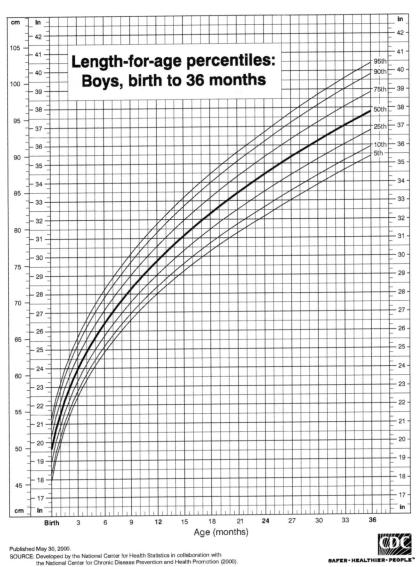

FIG. 16.10. Length-for-age percentiles: boys 0 to 36 months. (Developed by the National Center for Health Statistics in collaboration with the National Center for Chronic Disease.)

CDC Growth Charts: United States

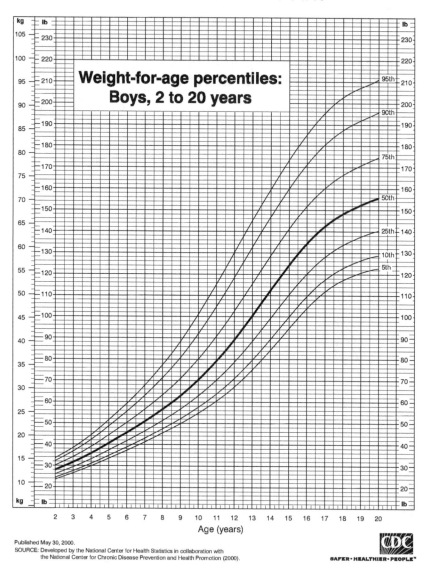

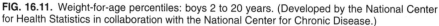

Published May 30, 2000.
SOURCE: Developed by the National Center for Health Statistics in collaboration with
the National Center for Chronic Disease Prevention and Health Promotion (2000).

FIG. 16.11. Weight-for-age percentiles: boys 2 to 20 years. (Developed by the National Center for Health Statistics in collaboration with the National Center for Chronic Disease.)

CDC Growth Charts: United States

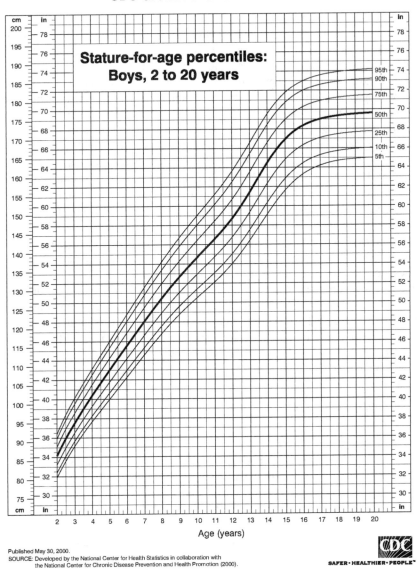

Published May 30, 2000.
SOURCE: Developed by the National Center for Health Statistics in collaboration with
the National Center for Chronic Disease Prevention and Health Promotion (2000).

FIG. 16.12. Stature-for-age percentiles: boys 2 to 20 years. (Developed by the National Center for Health Statistics in collaboration with the National Center for Chronic Disease.)

Identify Growth Patterns

Patterns of growth can be important indicators of risk for overweight and obesity. Although birth weight is largely dependent on maternal weight, newborns who are large for gestational age with a maternal history of diabetes or gestational diabetes are at increased risk for obesity and require close attention in achieving optimal energy balance. Conversely, newborns who are small for gestational age or who are from pregnancies complicated by cigarette smoking or other risk factors for intrauterine growth retardation, are also at increased risk for obesity and require close monitoring of growth.

In a study of California children under the age of 5, it was found that 39% of children from birth to 6 months of age, 6% to 15% of children between 6 and 24 months of age, and 1% to 5% of children 24 to 60 months of age crossed two major weight-for-age percentiles. Even more striking, 62% of children from birth to 6 months of age crossed two major weight-for-height percentiles, with 80% moving to higher percentiles. In addition, 20% to 27% of children 6 to 24 months of age and 8% to 15% of children 24 to 60 months of age crossed two major BMI-for-age percentiles About 14.5% of children between ages 2 and 3 years crossed two major BMI percentiles, down to 10.6% by age 4 years and 8.4% by age 5 years (1).

When it is determined that a child has crossed growth percentiles on the BMI chart, it is often useful to ask the family and child about any health, environmental, family, or psychosocial events that may have occurred around the time of the increase in BMI (Table 16.1). Although you may not always be able to identify inciting events, frequently this type of history gives you a glimpse of possible trigger points in the individual child and family that may have altered energy balance.

Identify children at risk for obesity between the 85th and 95th percentiles of BMI.

CHILDREN WITH BODY MASS INDEX BETWEEN THE 85TH AND 95TH PERCENTILES

Family History Focused on Obesity-Related Comorbidities

At this point, a family history of obesity and obesity-related comorbidities should be obtained if not done previously and can be used as a starting point for discussion with the family and child. For example, a family concerned about type 2 diabetes and complications in a grandparent can give information about the links to weight

TABLE 16.1. *Trigger points that may be associated with an increase in body mass index*

Parental separation/divorce	School change
Death of family member	Child's illness or hospitalization
Parental illness	Change in caregivers
Onset of depression	Family move

and lifestyle as well as be given a chance to express their concerns if this topic is introduced in a way that avoids blame and guilt. Parents, grandparents, siblings, and extended family may have had these conditions identified or may be having symptoms of the comorbidities outlined in Table 16.2.

If the family history is positive for familial hyperlipidemia or if parents or grandparents have had coronary atherosclerosis, myocardial infarction, angina pectoris, peripheral vascular disease, cerebrovascular disease, or sudden cardiac death or stroke at age 55 years or younger or cholesterol levels higher than 240 mg/dL, lipid screening should be performed. Factors such as diabetes, physical inactivity, cigarette smoking, and extended family with cardiovascular disease also contribute to risk and would indicate screening (2). A fasting plasma glucose should be obtained and repeated every 2 years if a child has a BMI greater than the 85th percentile and is 10 years old or has had onset of puberty with a family history of type 2 diabetes in parents, siblings, or grandparents; is of nonwhite race; has acanthosis nigricans; or has hypertension, dyslipidemia, or polycystic ovary syndrome (3).

Behavioral Changes

It is important to remember that physicians can have a direct impact on behavior changes. Literature on smoking cessation would suggest that assessment of patient readiness to quit smoking and provision of information on smoking cessation strategies in a primary care office can result in an increased number of patients who stop smoking (4). It is also important to note that in a study of overweight and obese children and adolescents from the National Health and Nutrition Examination Survey (NHANES) 1999–2000 only 36.7% of overweight children and adolescents ages 2 to 19 report being told by their physician or any health care provider that they were overweight. Children or their parents were more likely to be told they were overweight at older ages, with 17.4% of 2 to 5 year olds, 32.6% of 6 to 11 year olds, 39.6% of 12 to 15 year olds, and 51.6% of 16 to 19 year olds being told they were overweight (5).

IDENTIFY CHILDREN WITH BODY MASS INDEX GREATER THAN THE 95TH PERCENTILE

Children with BMI greater than the 95th percentile need evaluation and treatment for obesity. It goes without saying that the earlier in the obesity trajectory children

TABLE 16.2. *Family history of obesity-related comorbidities*

Obesity	Liver disease (NASH)
Sleep apnea	Polycystic ovarian syndrome
Asthma	Slipped capital femoral epiphysis
Gastroesophageal reflux	Blount's disease
Type 2 diabetes	Osteoarthritis
Hypertension	Cancer
Dyslipidemia	

NASH, nonalcoholic steatohepatitis.

are identified, the more time is available to integrate lifestyle and behavioral change. Family history in this group of children is also a good starting point for discussion. In addition, a thorough review of systems for obesity-related comorbidities should be carried out (Table 16.3).

TABLE 16.3. *Review of systems for obesity-related comorbidities and obesity-associated conditions*

Severe obesity-related emergencies
Cardiomyopathy of obesity
  Shortness of breath, orthopnea, dyspnea on exertion, pedal edema, rales, cardiomegaly
Diabetic ketoacidosis, hyperosmolar hyperglycemic state
  Polyuria, polydipsia, recent weight loss, blurred vision, abdominal pain, vomiting, vaginitis, prolonged infection, acanthosis nigricans, stupor, coma
Pulmonary emboli
  Recent immobilization, lower extremity surgery, chest pain, dyspnea, hypoxia

Obesity-related comorbidities requiring immediate attention
Slipped capital femoral epiphysis
  Hip, knee, or thigh pain; limp; uneven, painful gait
Blount's disease
  Tibial bowing; uneven, painful gait
Pseudotumor cerebri
  Headache, vomiting, papilledema, visual field cuts
Nonalcoholic steatohepatitis
  Anorexia, abdominal discomfort, hepatomegaly
Cholelithiasis
  Right upper quadrant pain, jaundice, vomiting

Chronic obesity-related comorbidities
Type 2 diabetes
  Polyuria, polydipsia, recurrent infections, vaginitis, recent weight loss, blurred vision
Asthma
  Shortness of breath, exercise-induced wheezing or cough
Obstructive sleep apnea syndrome
  Snoring, apnea, upright sleep position, daytime somnolence, poor school performance
Polycystic ovarian syndrome
  Acne, hirsutism, irregular menstrual periods or oligomenorrhea, acanthosis nigricans, history of premature adrenarche
Dyslipidemia
  Acanthosis nigricans, family history of lipid disorder
Hypertension
  Headache, systolic and/or diastolic blood pressure greater than the 90th percentile for age and gender
Depression
  Poor school performance, depressed affect, family history of depression, anger/behavioral issues
Binge eating disorder
  Out of control eating, sneaking, and guilt after eating
Bulimia
  Erosion of dental enamel, history of self-induced vomiting
Prader-Willi syndrome
  Neonatal hypotonia, small hands and feet, hyperphagia, skin picking, hypogonadism, developmental delay
Bardet-Biedl syndrome
  Polydactyly, renal anomalies, retinitis pigmentosa, developmental delay
MC4R mutations
  Severe childhood obesity and polyphagia

Screening

Screening laboratory studies should include a fasting lipid profile (2,6). Screening for type 2 diabetes also should be performed. Fasting glucose and insulin levels have been recommended (7), as are liver function studies (8). Other laboratory evaluation and further testing are based on the family history, review of systems, and physical examination.

Identify Children with Elevated Body Mass Index and Short Stature or Height Deceleration

Children with elevated BMI and short stature or height deceleration need immediate attention. These children should be evaluated for associated findings consistent with central nervous system (CNS) tumor (9) or hypothalamic lesion (10,11). History of hypothalamic injury; irradiation or surgery; genetic syndrome; endocrinologic disorders such as Cushing's syndrome, hypothyroidism, or growth hormone deficiency; or other systemic illnesses or pharmacologic treatment should also be addressed.

Evaluation of these children should include appropriate endocrinologic, genetic, and neurologic imaging studies and referral to a pediatric neurologist, geneticist, and/or endocrinologist.

It is important to remember that obese children and adolescents have the same needs for preventive care, ongoing health care, mental health services, and attention to behavioral issues as normal weight children, in addition to the increased risk conferred by obesity. It is vital to discuss obesity-related issues and problems in the context of overall well and illness-related care.

Treatment

Once a child is identified as obese, energy balance must be re-established. Initial goals for therapy can vary, depending on the magnitude of the obesity, the comorbidities that are present, and the age of the child. Table 16.4 illustrates categories of potential initial therapeutic goals.

It is important to identify the medical goals and outcome but to remember that the pathway to achieving these goals and restoring energy balance is individual, and

TABLE 16.4. *Potential initial therapeutic goals*

Slowing of rate of weight gain
Stabilizing weight
Reducing weight
Restoring metabolic parameters to normal
Reducing or eliminating obesity-related comorbidities
Changing targeted nutrition or activity behavior
Instituting family-based change
Improving the nutritional/activity environment

goals for lifestyle change should be set in collaboration with the family, based on their motivation, skills, and resources. A good review of strategies for achieving weight control is outlined by Dietz and Robinson (12), whose summary of weight control strategies include the following:

- Goal setting
- Control of the environment
- Monitoring and rewarding successful behavior
- Problem solving and parenting skills

Goal Setting

Goal setting (12) is achieved jointly with the family. Goals are based on detailed knowledge of the child's or adolescent's:

- Daily nutrition
- Activity and inactivity routine
- The family's approach to nutrition and activity
- Child's temperament
- Parenting style
- Parental and family belief that change can occur
- Value for the outcome of the behavior change

The role of the pediatrician and primary care physician is to provide sound medical evaluation of the child's current risk for disease, offer a menu of strategies that have proven effective in weight control based on the child's developmental stage, and work with the child and family to achieve these goals.

Goals should be **short term,** that is, what will happen by the next visit, and measurable, that is, minutes of outdoor play per day.

Goals should be **achievable.** Many families want to change every aspect of nutrition all at once, or have the adolescent "lose 50 lb by the prom."

Reassurance that stepwise change is effective and tends to be more long lasting is important to avoid setting up a situation of repeated failure.

Goals should be **family oriented.** Whenever possible, the whole family should participate in the behavioral change. For example, if television and computer use is being limited, this applies to the whole family, not just the obese child or adolescent. This strategy creates a partnership between the child and family and can limit the child's feeling of deprivation or resentment.

Goals should be **incremental.** Change is difficult under the best of circumstances. Setting one or two goals at a time can help solidify change and create stable habits to build on. Families should be reassured that you will partner with them as long as it takes to achieve weight control and good health for their child.

Control of the Environment

Control of the environment (12) is a strategy that focuses the family on the external environment and removes the intense focus some families have on the obese child. It may be helpful to compare the creation of an optimal nutritional and activity environment for the child with the time when the family "child proofed the house" for safety reasons. It can also be useful to help the family members see themselves as the interface between the child and the societal environment, which is obesity promoting. Families can begin to see that changing the home environment and helping the child or adolescent make healthy decisions about the nutritional and activity environment outside the home is a major teaching role for the adults in the family. Some environmental changes that have been found useful in weight control and in achieving healthy energy balance are listed in Table 16.5.

Self-Monitoring and Problem Solving

Setbacks are a normal part of lifestyle change.

TABLE 16.5. *Environmental changes to restore healthy energy balance*

Engage entire family in the desired environmental change

Limit availability of highly palatable, calorie-dense foods
Limit or eliminate juice, soda, sports drinks, and calorie-containing beverages (13)
Replace high-calorie snack food with healthy food choices that complete the food group requirements, such as fruits and vegetables
Eliminate "unconscious eating," i.e., eating in front of the television or computer, and instead have snacks and meals at the table

Increase meal structure
Have regular meal and snack times; avoid grazing and late night eating
Serve age-appropriate portions
Limit eating out and ordering in meals

Limit sedentary activity
Limit television and computer use to no more than 2 hours/day; no television or computer for children younger than 2 years (14)
Choose day care and after school care settings that provide activity opportunities when possible
Plan family activities around physical activity instead of sedentary behavior
Limit stroller use in toddler-aged child
Increase physical activity
Provide opportunity and time for outdoor play
Encourage parents to value extracurricular sports as opportunities for participation, not only competition
Help parents choose a variety of sport and physical activities to expand the child's and adolescent's physical repertoire
Increase the physical component of daily activities, e.g., park farther away from stores, walk from school or bus stop

Reprinted from Dietz WH, Robinson TN. Clinical practice: overweight children and adolescents. *N Engl J Med.* 2005; 352(20):2100–2109, with permission.

Preparing parents and family members in advance to expect some setbacks is helpful in sustaining change. Offering to be a partner in problem solving can relieve anxiety when setbacks occur. Building self-monitoring skills in conjunction with problem solving allows behavioral and lifestyle change to be maintained over time. Problem solving can be targeted to the specific goals that have been agreed on—for example, if the family decided to eliminate soda and juice from the house but the child gets sweetened drinks at grandmother's house after school, a family meeting that includes grandmother might be helpful to reset goals and develop a strategy to achieve them that whole family can support. Table 16.6 illustrates some common setbacks or problems that can arise in implementing a weight control plan (12).

Parenting Style and Skills

By definition, making behavioral change involves a close interaction between family members, parents, and the child or adolescent. Initiating change may trigger behavior in the child or adolescent that parents need to respond to, may cause friction between family members, and may necessitate an examination of parenting skills and style (12).

Communication

- Parents or responsible adults in charge need to agree on and be willing to participate in the desired behavior change.
- Desired changes need to be communicated to the child and family in a clear, authoritative, but not authoritarian, manner.
- Self-monitoring and frequent feedback needs to be communicated between the parent and child.
- Communication should be positive, with praise for success and a neutral and helpful approach when there are setbacks.
- Discussion about food, television, and computer should be limited to desired change, and the focus should be on the other areas of the child's life, such as friends, school, and family, to avoid overfocusing the parent-child communication on one area.

TABLE 16.6. *Common setbacks and problems*

Family members disagreeing on nutrition and activity changes
Child or adolescent getting extra meals, snacks, and food at school, day care, relatives and friends, and corner store
Free access to food after school
Family schedule that interferes with meal timing and structure
Television and computer in child's room, multiple televisions in house
Limited availability of resources for physical activity, limited knowledge of community resources

Setting Boundaries

- Parents need to see themselves as providers of good nutrition and children and adolescents as deciders of how much of the correct portion to eat.
- Parents can think of nutrition and activity decisions as health decisions in the same way they think of decisions about safety. This may help them maintain boundaries in the face of resistance.
- It is appropriate for parents to encourage participation in physical activities in the same way they support the child's success at school and with other extracurricular activities.
- Parents are the gatekeepers in terms of environmental, societal, and cultural influences on eating and activity and should decide how they want to maintain healthy behaviors rather than adopting the norm.

Setting Examples

- Parents and responsible adults should behave in the same way they would like the child or adolescent to behave, even if they do not have a weight problem.
- Parents should examine their own lifestyle choices and be willing to change if necessary.
- Parents can model ways of dealing with problems and setbacks.
- Parents can model optimal communication around the often emotionally charged issues of eating and physical activity change.

PRACTICE-BASED CHANGE

To help patients and families affected by and at risk for obesity, practices will have to change workflow to incorporate this "new work of pediatrics." In many ways, the same principles for making behavior change in families apply to making change in practice.

Possible Practice-Based Strategies to Consider

Timing

It is important to decide how the practice will incorporate obesity-related issues into the visit schedule. Some possibilities include the following:

- **Prenatal visit**

> Breastfeeding should be encouraged as the optimal nutrition source for all infants but has also been shown to have a small but significant effect on later obesity (15).

Parental obesity is a risk for childhood and adolescent obesity, and families in which one or both parents are obese can be identified and supported in assessing family nutrition and activity patterns as early as possible (16).

- **Well visits**

Establish a routine of plotting height, weight, and BMI and reviewing growth with parents at every well visit. A quick diet and activity history can target areas for discussion of optimal nutrition and activity habits. Establishing a routine review will normalize the discussion about BMI for parents.

- **Illness-related visits**

A visit relating to a comorbidity of obesity can also be an opportunity to briefly assess progress on lifestyle change or to suggest a follow-up visit to continue work on weight control.

Tracking

Once a child is identified as obese or at risk for obesity, the practice should have a routine for scheduling revisits to initiate treatment and track progress. It is helpful to have all practitioners agree to a similar routine in assessing and treating obesity so families experience a consistent approach to this problem.

Triggers

Children whose BMI is between the 85th and 95th percentiles, children with a BMI greater than the 95th percentile, and children crossing growth percentiles should trigger an evaluation of family history, review of systems, laboratory testing, identification of any obesity-related comorbidities, and a plan for follow-up visits.

Emergencies

Staff education should include information about obesity-related emergencies and comorbidities, including signs and symptoms, and a plan of action.

REFERENCES

1. Mei Z, Grummer-Strawn LM, Thompson D, Dietz WH. Shifts in percentiles of growth during early childhood; analysis of longitudinal data from the California Child Health and Development study. *Pediatrics.* 2004;113:e617–e627 (accessed 8/12/06 at http://pediatrics.aappublications.org/cgi/content/full/113/6/e617/F3).
2. American Academy of Pediatrics Committee on Nutrition. Cholesterol in childhood. *Pediatrics.* 1998;101:141–147.
3. American Diabetes Association. Type 2 diabetes in children and adolescents. *Diabetes Care.* 2000; 105(3Pt1):671–680.
4. Milch CE, Edmunson JM, Beshansky JR, Griffith JL, Selker HP. Smoking cessation in primary care: a clinical effectiveness trial of two simple interventions. *Prev Med.* 2004;38:284–294.
5. Ogden CL, Tabak CJ. Children and teens told by doctors that they were overweight–United States, 1999–2002. *MMWR.* 2005;54(34):848–849.

6. Bao W, Srinivasan SR, Wattigney WE, Bao W, Berencon GS. Usefulness of childhood low-density lipoprotein cholesterol level in predicting adult dyslipidemia and other cardiovascular risks. The Bogalusa Heart Study. *Arch Intern Med.* 1996;156:1315–1320.
7. Barlow SE, Dietz WH. Obesity evaluation and treatment: Expert Committee recommendations. The Maternal and Child Health Bureau, Health Resources and Services Administration and the Department of Health and Human Services. *Pediatrics.* 1998;102(3):e29.
8. Strauss RS, Barlow SE, Dietz WH. Prevalence of abnormal serum aminotransferase values in overweight and obese adolescents. *J Pediatr.* 2000;136(6):727–733.
9. Muller HL, Emser A, Faldum A, Bruhnken G, Etavard-Gorris, N, Gebhardt U, Oeverink R, Kolb R, Sorensen N. Longitudinal study on growth and body mass index before and after diagnosis of childhood craniopharyngioma. *J Clin Endocrinol Metab.* 2004;98:3298–3305.
10. Cianfarani S, Nicholl RM, Medbach S, Charlesworth MC, Savage MO. Idiopathic hypothalamus pituitary dysfunction: review of five cases. *Horm Res.* 1993;39(1–2):47–50.
11. Mehta S, Boyd T, Weinstein D. Ganglioneuroblastoma in children with rapid weight gain and obesity: an infrequently recognized paraneoplastic syndrome. Abstract International Endocrine Meetings, Lyon, France, 2005.
12. Dietz WH, Robinson TN. Clinical practice: overweight children and adolescents. *N Engl J Med.* 2005;352(20):2100–2109.
13. Berkey CS, Rockett HR, Field AE, Gillman MW, Colditz GA. Sugar-added beverages and adolescent weight change. *Obes Res.* 2004;12:778–788.
14. American Academy of Pediatrics. Children, adolescents and television. Committee on Public Education. *Pediatrics.* 2001;107:423–426.
15. Harder T, Bergmann R, Kallischnigg G, Plagemann A. Duration of breastfeeding and risk of overweight: a meta analysis. *Am J Epidemiol.* 2005;162:397–403.
16. Whitaker RC, Wright JA, Pep MS, Seidel KD, Dietz WH. Predicting obesity in young adulthood from childhood and parental obesity. *N Engl J Med.* 1997;337:869–873.

Index

Note: Page numbers in *italics* indicate figures and page numbers followed by "t" indicate tables concerning the subject.